The Evolution Diet

What and How We Were Designed to Eat

Joseph Stephen Breese Morse

Edited by E. Robert Morse

The Evolution Diet. Copyright © 2005 by Joseph Stephen Breese Morse. All Rights Reserved. Printed in the United States of America. No part of this book may be used or reproduced in any manner whatsoever without written consent by the author. Exceptions are granted for brief quotations within critical articles or reviews.

Amelior Publishing is an imprint of CoDe Publishing.
For information address CoDe Publishing, PO 928483, San Diego, CA, 92192-8483.

Designed by Code Interactive (www.code-interactive.com)

ISBN 1 60020 0389

*To Kathleen, Alyson, Eric, and Mum.
Whether agreeing or challenging,
it was always support. Thanks.*

Contents

Part One: The Evolution Diet — 1
    An Introduction — 1
    Was It Something I Ate? — 2
    Background of the Diet — 5
    A Brief Explanation of the Diet — 6
    The Purpose of A Diet — 9

Part Two: The Way We Evolved — 15
    Oral Cavity — 17
    Digestive Tract — 18
    How A Dynamic Physiology Helps Humans — 22

Part Three: The Cultureless Diet — 25
    Cultural Influences — 27
    Personal Influences — 29
    What A Cultureless Human Would Eat — 32

Part Four: The Body's Chemistry — 37
    Carbohydrate Is Not A Four Letter Word — 38
    What's In a Carb? — 39
    What Does Too Much Sugar Do To Us? — 43
    We Are Made of Protein — 46
    With Friends Like Fats, Who Needs Enemies? — 50

Part Five: Now We're Ready to Get Started!   55
    The Fundamentals   56
    Listen To Your Body   57
    Appropriate Your Diet   60
    Avoid Intake of Artificially Extreme Foods   63

Part Six: A Sample Diet   73
    What The Evolution Diet Looks Like   73

Part Seven: Other Factors   83
    Basal Metabolism   83
    Exercise When Your Body Tells You To   86
    The Origin Of Exercise   88
    The Importance Of Exercise   89
    Breathing And Sleep   91
    Stress   92

Part Eight: What You'll Get In Return   95
    Some Initial Side Effects   96
    Some Positive Things To Look For   97
    A Better Life   99

Part Nine: Everything Else   101
    Breakfast and LoS Hi-Fi foods List   102
    High-Protein Dinner Foods   106
    Energy Foods   112
    Calorie Expenditures of Various Exercises   116
    Recipes   119
        LoS Hi-Fi foods   119
        High-Protein Dinner Foods   139
    Glossary   167

Notes 173
Bibliography 174

Part One
The Evolution Diet
(An Introduction)

"The first thing dieters lose is their sense of humor."
-Anonymous

Get to and maintain your ideal weight. Feel healthy and energetic throughout the day. Sleep well every night. Do these things seem impossible for you? Does the idea of a truly healthy lifestyle seem so unlikely that you've almost given up? If that sounds like you, you've been listening to the wrong people. It's time to escape from the negative unhealthy lifestyle, and it's time to evolve into the person you were designed to be.

If you have ever been curious as to how your body works or why we eat the things we do, this is the book for you. You are about to embark on an educational, insightful, enlightening, and often humorous journey as you learn what, and *how*, your body is designed to eat.

For nearly two million years, humans were eating in the hunter/gatherer style of foraging for plants and then hunting for large game. Our bodies were uniquely designed, as we'll learn later, to eat in this manner. However, about 9000 years ago, humans started eating a different way. We learned agriculture and began our move to a sedentary, unhealthy lifestyle.

Recently humans have been paying the price for eating in a manner contrary to how we were designed. The skyrocketing obesity rates, ubiquitous prescription drugs, and persistent unhappiness throughout the population are signs that humans are not eating how they were designed. The Evolution Diet can help. It is a painstakingly developed, yet astonishingly easy-to-follow method of getting back to your natural, healthy self.

All you really need to do to become a healthier, happier person is to follow four principles: 1. Listen to your body, not your culture, 2. Appropriate your diet in the method of our ancestors, 3. Avoid intake of Artificially Extreme Foods (AEFs) like fried Twinkies, and 4. Exercise and sleep when your body tells you to. This seems simple, but not too many people in today's society do it. The Evolution Diet will explain how you can achieve your physical and emotional goals in easy, common sense steps.

Was It Something I Ate?

I'd like to begin with a story from a couple of our first trial dieters. It's possible that you will be able to identify with them as you learn of their trials through dieting. You can be assured that they have become avid Evolution Dieters and are now living refreshingly healthy lives.

Bob was one of the first to start the Evolution Diet. He had always pictured himself as a healthy person all his life, but his diet had consistently fluctuated dramatically. He had played sports and had been physically active for his entire adult life, rarely going a couple of days without exercise. However, he figured that since he was exercising, he could eat anything he wanted and in whatever manner pleased him. He went from eating large, fat-saturated Taco Bell lunches 4 times a week in high school, to eating absolutely nothing all day between breakfast and dinner. He would eat 4 course meals for brunch in college and on top of that, wolf down a full pizza at 3 A.M. after a night out!

Although Bob was active, probably more so than his average cohorts, he was not healthy. His diet was unbalanced and not nutritious, and the consequences were blatant. He was slightly overweight and had such inconsistent spurts of energy and fatigue that it was debilitating. Eventually, his sleep pattern was affected and he found himself, like 70% of Americans, suffering from sleep problems. He was tired at the wrong times of the day and restless at night. Exercising helped reduce the effects of the bad diet by helping reduce blood pressure and burning more calories than he would otherwise, but eating poorly deterred him from doing exercise and reduced his interest in doing it in the first place.

Hindsight is always 20/20, so it seems obvious that Bob could have been leading a much more productive and happy life if he had just paid a little attention to what he was eating. Eventually he dabbled in eating methods (he didn't want to call it a diet) that were supposed to make him healthier.

He didn't think there was a problem with his breakfast, but when we discussed his habits, he was shocked to discover he was eating extremely sugary foods and mass quantities of it accompanied with a large glass of orange juice (also very sugary). He figured there couldn't be anything wrong with orange juice since it was all natural, and the little crunchy cereal bits he was eating at least resembled fruit. Although he didn't make the connection, when he got to work after this meal and just sat at his desk, he was wired and irritable and couldn't focus. Was it that he couldn't handle sitting at a desk in an office all day, or was it that he wasn't eating well?

Our friend Bob is an experimental type and after acknowledging his unhealthiness, he decided to make changes in his diet to see if that would help him feel better. First, he focused on getting rid of the nasty vending machine food that he ate for lunch, and he replaced it with a 1300-calorie veggie burrito from Rojello's Mexican restaurant down the street. This bowling-ball-in-your-stomach-food-coma-after-lunch-diet, however appealing it may have seemed to Bob, did not work either.

Since that didn't work, he tried a second method to try to eat better and that was to eliminate all food after breakfast until he got home from work. This might seem crazy to some, but Bob was confounded at the fact that he exercised nearly every day, but was still slightly overweight. He wasn't like those challenged individuals who have to buy two airplane tickets to be comfortable flying, but he had about 10-15 extra pounds and it was uncomfortable for him. Bob was willing to try anything and at the time, the midday fast seemed like an okay idea.

Bob was proud of his diet at first. He said he probably lost some weight initially, but his energy was more inconsistent than ever and he felt like passing out by the end of the workday. Believe it or not, with such a decrease in caloric intake, Bob ended up gaining weight! Needless to say, this eating method didn't last very long.

Another current Evolution Dieter, Susan, had tried the high protein diet and its spin-offs, with some success in losing weight, but horrible failure in her attempts to feel better and more energetic. Susan figured the high protein diet, "was just boring me into weight loss. I could only eat certain things and after a while I didn't feel like eating those same things, so I ate less. Not to mention, I barely had enough energy to make it through a large steak after a couple months on the diet."

After that, she took a different approach: she had a small protein breakfast and a couple snacks around midday. These snacks tended to be extremely dense and highly sugary foods, mainly dried fruit trail mix and energy bars. Although Susan wasn't gaining any weight, she said it seemed like she was at an all time irritability high. In addition, when she didn't have food for any extended period, she would begin to shut down in a mild version of the condition termed hypoglycemia (low blood sugar).

Neither of these candidates, Bob or Susan, was healthy before the Evolution Diet, but they could not figure out why they were unhealthy considering they were both eating so-called "health foods." They got to the point where they were eating pretty much all natural foods, and both were eating moderate proportions with regard to hunger. They were not stuffing their faces, and only eating when they were hungry. They just could not figure out why they felt so unhealthy. This is when they decided to contact nutritional specialists and learn how to become truly healthy.

I took them on as studies and promoted what has become the Evolution Diet.

Background of the Diet

I began my study of how the human body should take in food around the year 2000. What I learned was shocking, however obvious it may seem after the fact: the modern American diet is dramatically

> **An Evolution Diet Essential:**
> This Diet is not just a way to lose weight quickly, but a plan for maintaining a perfectly healthy lifestyle for your entire life.

contrary to what we, as humans were designed to eat. I learned that institutions such as the "three square" and the "balanced meal" are actually bad for you. I learned that most of the foods in our diets have been so densely packed with ingredients that almost every time you eat, you are overloading your system, which causes detrimental stress on the bodily system.

I learned stunning facts that dispute current popular diets, such as the high protein diet. In that diet, authors will tell you that a slice of bread is full of empty and easily digested carbs, which will give you a spike in your blood sugar. The 'protein only' promoters would consider such a slice of bread equivalent to a can of sugary cola. I learned that this is dead wrong. The body takes in 30 calories a minute from the can of cola, but just 2 calories a minute from the bread! The two food items may have the same total calories, but the complex nature of the bread makes the digestion a great deal more balanced, and therefore healthier. These are the types of insight that you will gain with the Evolution Diet.

Through research and the study, I've developed a plan for eating which takes into account two factors of modern food variety and your very own natural processes. The Evolution Diet is not just a way to lose weight quickly, but also a plan for maintaining a perfectly healthy lifestyle for your entire life.

In addition, when you eat the way you were designed to eat, you will not only achieve your ideal weight, but you will feel energetic when you should, sleepy when it's time, and generally happy throughout the day. Sounds good doesn't it? The major problem with today's lifestyle is that we've gotten too far away from our natural diet, forcing the cultural constraints on our physiology. The results are scary: depression, sleeplessness, fatigue, and of course, obesity.

It's important to understand the effects of one's diet. Even for people who are not overweight, your diet is integral to your health. If you have been feeling inexplicable irritability, sadness, fatigue, loss in alertness, or just lack of good health, the latest pharmaceutical pill is NOT the answer! If you alter what you eat, and more importantly *how* you eat, just a bit, you will be on the way to living a perfectly healthy, and happy life. Take control again — you can do it!

A Brief Explanation of the Diet

The Evolution Diet is a revolutionary way of looking at what you eat. It encourages you to get more in touch with your body and know how it was designed to eat. It also encourages you to eat how you were meant to eat, not just what you were meant to eat. When this happens, you will eat the types of food you would without the influences of culture and regain the ideal weight you may have lost previously. This will lead to a happier, healthier life all around.

The amazing thing about the Evolution Diet is that it is a consistent plan for eating throughout your life. While most other diets start you off with a "shock-your-system" introduction followed by eating in moderation, the Evolution Diet calls for one life-long method of eating, which reflects your personal lifestyle and can support you through activity or inactivity.

> **An Evolution Diet Essential:**
> The goal is to imitate the diet of natural humans (those without out strong cultural influences) to fit the diet our bodies have been naturally designed for.

The goal is to imitate the diet of natural humans (or, as referred to later, Natural Man) in order to fit the diet our bodies have been designed to take. Regardless of how you think our species was designed, we are made to eat certain things and in a certain way. Natural Man (without present culture) had been around 500 times longer than Cultural Man and our overly efficient foods. During all that time, Natural Man developed a way to eat based on his surroundings and environment, which varies only slightly outside of the Arctic Circle. In essence, Natural Man evolved to eat a certain way.

He ate small quantities of low sugar, high fiber foods (explained later as LoS Hi-Fi foods) throughout the day until he hunted and subsequently gorged himself on mass quantities of nutritious meat. This simplified version of the subsistence hunter/gatherer shows a rough expectation of the foods our bodies are expecting us to feed it. If we don't feed it that diet, it reacts adversely with the conditions listed above.

If you enjoy eating, and most of us do, then you will enjoy this method. Most people eat more on this diet than they did before, yet they achieve their ideal weight and keep it off. A simple idea one must realize, however, is that eating is only enjoyable to humans because it originally helped us live. In our modern society, however, the food we eat is actually detrimental to our health. We did not evolve to eat fried Twinkies and 64 ounce Big Gulps.

Besides eating, we humans can entertain ourselves quite thoroughly. We can play games, sing, write poetry, build Channel Tunnels and Hoover Dams, and most importantly, we can educate our young. Eating should be seen as a means to do all of those other things, instead of an end. Eating should make our bodies happy, and, in turn, make our minds happy.

The Evolution Diet takes our current modern foods and puts them into a method of eating which makes our bodies happy. This book will describe that method and get you to that place.

I will describe what we are made of physically, which will give us clues as to what we should be eating. Then I will take a

Case Study: Morena
Age: 46 Goal: Weight loss

The most astonishing thing about the Evolution Diet to Morena was the fact that just by altering the time when she ate certain foods, she lost weight.

"I ate about the same amount of food I normally was eating, maybe even more, but I lost weight from eating all my carbs throughout the day and all my proteins at night. It was amazing to see the pounds drop from just that!"

Morena learned the most basic aspect to The Evolution Diet: not only is it important to eat healthy foods, it's important to eat certain foods at certain times.

There's a place for almost every type of food you can imagine in The Evolution Diet, but one must eat them at the appropriate time. For instance, Morena always had a craving for buttered popcorn. She would usually cook up a batch in the late evening, about an hour before sleep. What she didn't realize was that she was filling herself with mostly carbohydrates and fat and not using those calories immediately because she was going to sleep.

All of these extra calories went straight to her waistline as stored fat.

When she moved her popcorn 'meal' to the daytime, the weight came off almost immediately.

lighter, and often unappetizing look at why we eat what we do, and what a cultureless person would eat. It is vital for us to understand what goes on in our bodies, at least to some extent, so I will then describe our bodies' chemistry and how it reacts to the main food types: carbohydrates, proteins, and fats.

With all of the background information down, I will describe, in depth, the Evolution Diet, and what exactly you should be eating and how you should be eating to match your modern lifestyle, but more importantly, to match how you were designed to eat. The results will be evident in your life, but I will give you positive physical reactions to look for in the last section. First, though, I would like to contest the current notion of diet and explain what a diet really should be seen as.

The Purpose of a Diet

Ever since certain fad diets became popular in the eighties, the general conception of a 'diet' is viewed as a tool to help its participants lose a few pounds, then return to their usual eating methods. In other words, it is seen as a short term fix. This type of yo-yo eating habit is confusing, however appealing it may seem. Testimonials similar to, "I lost 50 pounds in 5 weeks!" to, "I dropped 15 pounds the first week!" lead to inaccurate interpretations of what a diet should be. If these people were to continue on their so called diet, they would be weightless within a couple years. Now that would be amazing!

The truth is, these diets, which cut out so much weight instantly, are actually just dehydrating the body. The weight lost is in water (and since the body is about 60% water, it is fairly easy to do). Inevitably, the 'contestants' on these 'miracle diets' must change their habits back or at least alter them so as not to eliminate themselves from existence. Yet, a diet, by definition, is not some two week panacea to help you lose weight. A diet is someone's general intake of food. A diet is something that takes place over one's entire life, not just the five weeks before one's wedding day.

Changing one's eating habits so drastically is extremely unhealthy, something that most diet promoters fail to explain. An obese person has a better chance of living longer than someone who fluctuates often between being obese and having an ideal weight. <u>Health Day</u> has cited a University of Michigan report that has found a direct link to the gain-loss-gain syndrome of yo-yo dieting and cardiovascular disease in women.

That isn't to say that one shouldn't try to lose weight. Of course, the constantly obese person has a drastically small chance of living longer than someone at an ideal weight constantly. A Dutch study published in the <u>Annals of Internal Medicine</u> (2003) says that obese women live an average of 7.1 fewer years than women of normal weight. Obese men live 5.8 fewer years on average than their healthy counterparts. That's almost 10% of an average life!

The solution for everyone would be a method of eating which would bring everyone to their ideal weight and keep them there without going back and forth with different so-called diets. The common opposition to that statement would be, "Well, everyone is different. There can't possibly be a diet that works for everyone." That is one of the great aspects of the Evolution Diet: it supports a healthy lifestyle for everyone, regardless of physical makeup. Because this method of eating is strictly linked to the natural methods of the body, it will work to create a stable, healthy weight for everyone who adheres to the guidelines. One of the most integral concepts of the Evolution Diet is that it is even beneficial for people with ideal weights, thus someone can maintain just one diet for their entire life, the healthy way it should be.

What about the fat gene? Some people would argue that some people were born with a 'fat gene,' and it is nearly impossible for those people to maintain a healthy weight without surgery or medical assistance in the form of pills.

It is understandable if you have accepted this train of thought since it is everywhere in the popular media. There are people out there that want to make you think that *you* have no say in *your* physical state, but *their* magical pill does. That seems a little suspect to me.

It just so happens that there is very little, with respect to genes, that differs between humans, even when it comes to weight maintenance. A recent study conducted by Dr. Roy J. Britten at the California institute of Technology (published in Proceedings of the National Academy of Sciences) has found that even humans and chimpanzees have nearly identical genetic makeup. According to the study, 95% of the genetic make-up of chimps is the same as that of humans. Shockingly, we're even quite similar to a pumpkin. Similar methods of experimentation showed that pumpkins and humans share 75% of our DNA. However, this doesn't mean we need to look like a pumpkin! Based on these findings it appears that just being alive accounts for so much of our genetic code, that there is very little left over to produce differences like eating tendencies. The CIT study has found that two different humans are 99.9% genetically identical.

> **An Evolution Diet Essential:**
> Regardless of one's genetic makeup, everyone can be lean and fit. No one is precluded from attaining a healthy body and a healthy mind (with an ideal weight).

Based on the number of genes scientists have found that humans have (about 30,000), you are only 30 or so genes different from Mick Jagger. That's astounding. This applies to everyone with the normal amount of 23 paired chromosomes.

It turns out that our previous idea of a gene for every protein created was the wrong way to think about it. It's not the number of genes that determines what we are, but what our genes do with what they are given that gives us the diversity and complexity of being human. So we can actually alter what our genes do and how they work based on what we feed them. In other words we actually *are* what we eat.

Likewise, the perception that people have that their genetic makeup is what determines who they are is also false. It is what we DO with our genetic makeup that makes us who we are.

This stirs up the ancient argument of Nature versus Nurture, which to my knowledge has not been definitively answered. No one can deny we are products of our genes—just think of all the times you've heard, "You've got your father's eyes," or more unfortunately, "You've got your father's bald patch." But even the most ardent Naturalists will concede that behavior plays a significant role in one's construction. They would add that all people could be fit and healthy, though they would argue that some people need to try harder than others. I contest that it's not a matter of trying harder, but rather being more thoughtful and simply living how we were designed to live. Thus, without going in to the argument of Nature versus Nurture, we must stipulate that regardless of one's genetic make-up, everyone can be lean and fit. No one is precluded from attaining a healthy body and a healthy mind (with an ideal weight).

This is one of the most important factors in achieving a healthy lifestyle: You must know that you can do it for it to be possible at all. The beneficial aspects of positive psychology are unlimited, and though the idea is important to understand, it deserves its own book and I can't do it justice here. Instead, here's a list of clichés that illustrate positive thinking:

- "You can't achieve anything without trying."
- "A negative attitude will get you nowhere."
- "The luckiest people tend to be the one who always work harder."
- "Nothing valuable comes without a price."
- "Haste makes waste."
- "When life gives you lemons, make lemonade."
- "Turn that frown upside down." (This one doesn't really apply, but it's nice anyway)

Having said that, it is easier to understand that everyone is the same, more or less. I've heard countless times people say that it is impossible to be as thin as a supermodel, or some famous skinny actress. In fact, it is extremely probable based on another simple fact: if someone expends more calories than they take it, they will lose weight, and if someone takes in more calories than they burn, they will gain weight. This applies to the person behind the counter at the grocery store as much as it applies to Cindy Crawford or Gisele Bundchen. What these people mean to say when they say that, "It's impossible to be as thin as those models while eating what I eat and exercising as little as I do." That seems kind of obvious, doesn't it?

> **An Evolution Diet Essential:**
> There is a middle ground in weight at which the human body is perfectly content. It is a natural state of being, in which the calories ingested are equivalent to the calories expended and which there is no excess fat. This is the goal.

It is important to note that the idea here is not to be thin; in fact, super-thin supermodels are probably not as healthy as they could be, as some fat is necessary for a completely healthy body to operate (we will discuss this later). The important thing is to be healthy, which certainly includes not being overweight, but also includes not being underweight. There are equally detrimental problems associated with being underweight as there are with being overweight, although, in today's American society, the former is not as popular of a problem. It is also common to maintain a constant body weight while exercising and eating proportionally, yet, to still have an unhealthy body weight.

There is a middle ground in weight at which the human body is perfectly content. It is a natural state of being, in which the calories ingested are equivalent to the calories expended and which there is no excess storage of calories to maintain. This is the state that we should want to achieve. A state that is free from culturally influenced abnormalities like the three square meals, the gigantisized portions, Atkins, the celery diet, and fast food. This is a state of being which your body has been begging you to get to for all of your life. Your body has told you when you are not treating it right with uncomfortable feelings, guilt and, even pain.

It is time that you get to the state of perfect balance within yourself, start listening to your body and become the healthy individual you know you can be. It is time to evolve.

Part Two
How We Evolved
(The Omnivore Debate)

Q: What do you call a fake noodle?
A: AN IMPASTA.

"You know you are dieting when stamps start to taste good."
-Anonymous

    Human beings are quite the survivor species. We've been able to expand prolifically from a group of about 40,000 in Central Africa, to over 6 billion covering the entire globe. We have acclimated to most of the climates on Earth: barren deserts in the Americas to the bitter cold tundra of Northern Asia. We have been able to survive where other animals could not (forest, savannah, and mountains) and we're able to sit at the top of the food chain despite our species' lack of natural defense mechanisms, like claws.

    The human being is truly the most remarkable thing that is, or at least that we know about. One of the reasons we have been so successful in dominating our surroundings and rocketing to the top of the food chain is because of our large brain size. We are smart enough to catch larger animals, or to find fruits and vegetables that other animals cannot. So, a large portion of credit for our success should go to whoever thought of giving us a large brain. That was a good idea!

Besides being smart, though, we have other traits and abilities that make it possible for us to be so physically successful. Humans have things such as sharp canines, which may not seem like much, but allows us to chew meat so that we may more easily get to the proteins that our bodies need. Vegetarians will instantly refute this as an archaic remnant of a barbarous path of mammalian existence: the carnivore. But the teeth needed to cut meat and the acids in our stomachs exist in humans so that we may easily eat meat. What we should do with those traits now are up for debate.

In addition, we have a digestive system that, like it or not, contains billions of little helper animals which help break down foods to give us the nutrients that we need. Bacteria have a gigantic role in our digestion. Without the thousands of different types of bacterial living in our bodies, we would not be able to live. We are lucky that our bodies have chosen to be nice and allow those bacteria to remain in the Small Intestine Hotel and live instead of trying to kill them off like malicious intruders.

Another nice feature we have is our single stomach, which helps us maintain a relatively small abdomen and allows us to walk upright, instead of requiring four legs to hold us up. A cow has 4 different chambers in their stomach system. This is what's needed to digest the food they eat (mainly grass). Can you image having to walk around with 75 gallons of additional stomach space in your body? Not to mention having to regurgitate food that we've already eaten just to chew it back up and send it back through. We are lucky to have our one stomach, which can break up almost anything it comes in contact with.

All of these features that the human body has leads to one result: the ability to eat a wide variety of foods efficiently. Before explaining why this is a benefit to us as animals, I will describe the omnivore debate and explain why we are naturally omnivorous. In the class mammalia, there are vegetarians and meat-eaters. Which one of those we are naturally has been a matter of debate since the beginning of history. The most common name for humans is omnivore. However, many plant-eaters and strict meat-eaters among us have tried very hard to convince people that that name is inappropriate.

In determining whether an animal is herbivorous (strictly plant eating), frugivorous (mainly fruit eating), carnivorous (strictly meat eating), or omnivorous (eats just about anything), it is important to discern between effecting methods of logic, and otherwise. It is not good enough to say that humans are omnivorous because you see people eat a salad before dinner and a steak for dinner. Observation doesn't make for a complete study. I've seen a human being eat metal nails and screws, but that doesn't quite make it natural, healthy, or especially logical.

Many types of eating habits result in or from distinct physical characteristics. Using the physical characteristics that humans have and comparing those with the characteristics of animals in each eating type, we should be able to divulge the answer to the question: what should we be eating?

Oral Cavity

For most carnivores (picture your dog, Spot), the oral cavity, or mouth, is wide with spaced-out teeth, so as to prevent the stringy things from sticking around and prevent the times when we would use floss to get at them. The incisors are short and prong-like. They are used to grip onto prey. The canines are long and dagger like, used to stab and tear flesh. When the jaw of a carnivore closes, the teeth in the back come together like a pair of scissors in order to produce an effective cutting action.

Herbivores, on the other hand, don't need such cutting and slicing; tearing and stabbing. A herbivore's prey is pretty defenseless, because their prey is plant life. All an herbivore needs to get food in its stomach is a grinding mechanism. Herbivores' teeth are flatter and do not slide past one another to create a scissor-like cutting action. Some herbivores, like pigs, have enormous canines. These are most likely not used for hunting prey, but rather as a defense mechanism. Some herbivores may not even have canines, or just a bottom pair, as in the case of our friendly cow.

One important difference between most carnivores and most herbivores is the composition of their saliva. In most herbivores, there is an enzyme that aids in the digestion of carbohydrates, so that food digestion starts happening once the animal takes a bite. Carnivores, on the other hand, do not produce this enzyme. They wait for the food to get to their stomach to start digestion. This doesn't take very long when the carnivore is good at what it does. When the meat-eater kills prey it gorges itself and retreats away from the battleground to digest. Herbivores, like elephants aren't going to be hurried by anyone, since their food is so abundant and not difficult to capture. They can take their time and grind up their food right where they found it.

Digestive Tract

The differences between carnivores and herbivores with regard to their digestive tract are far more reaching and elaborate. To begin, carnivores have one stomach and very low pH level inside of it (around pH 1). This means that the environment in a carnivore's stomach is very acidic. The intensely acidic mixture of chemicals is needed to break apart the proteins in the meat. Additionally, the acid is used to kill off the detrimental bacteria, which thrive on flesh open to the air. The stomach in most carnivores is widely expandable in order to allow for large quantities of food in short amounts of time. Also, the small intestine is substantially shorter in carnivores.

Herbivores, as mentioned before may have multiple stomachs, which are needed for the longer digestion of the plants they eat. Strict herbivores (bovines for instance) have stomach capacities 150 times that of an average human's. The food sits in the digestive tract for longer amounts of time. To fully break down the cells in grass, for instance, to obtain the intracellular goodies,

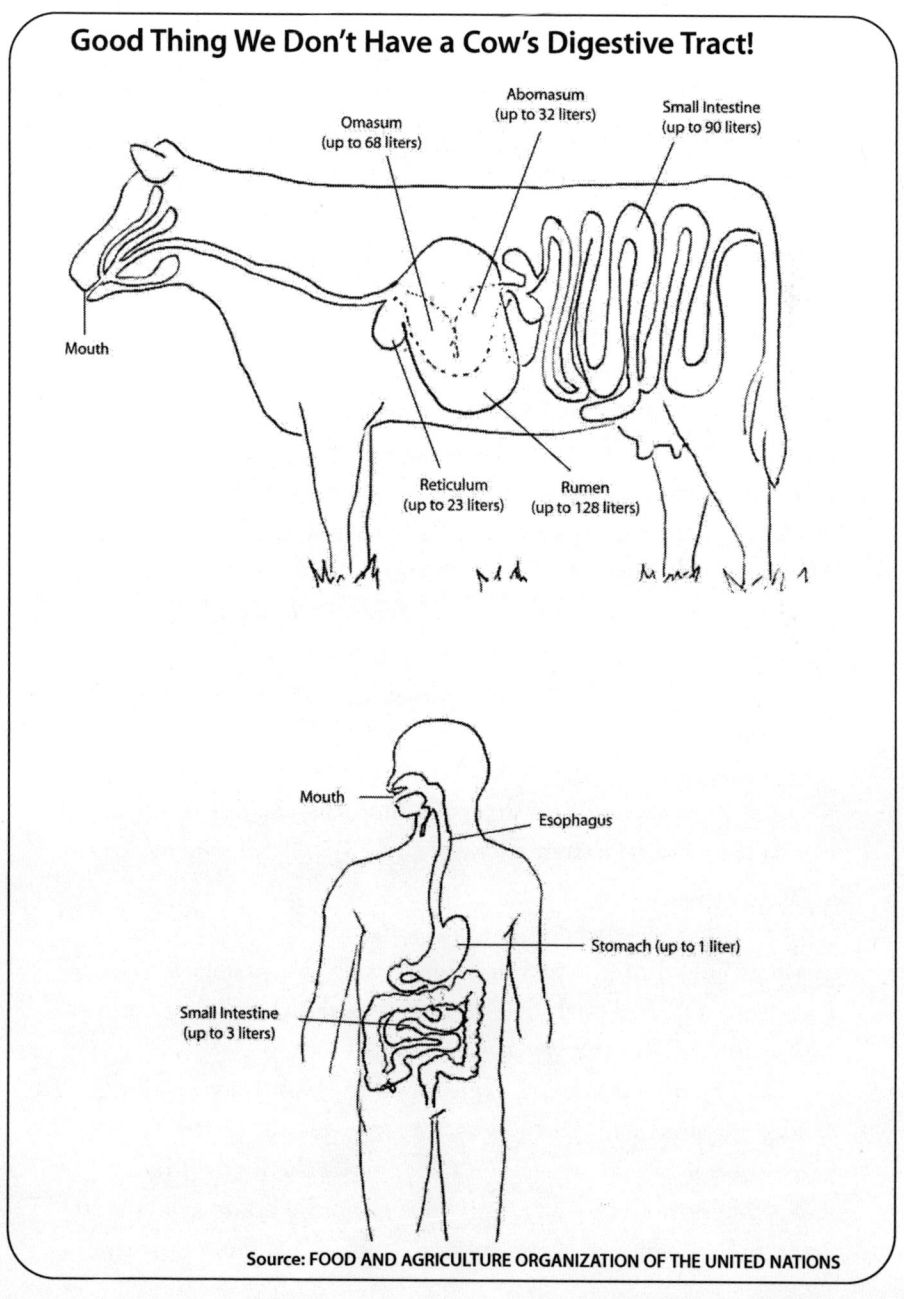

herbivores must let the mass of plants ferment in their digestive tract. This process of fermentation occurs when bacteria breaks down the substance for the host animal. Many herbivores do not ferment cellulose (the fiber found in much of plant life), for they eat more easily digested soft vegetation, things like fruits and vegetables.

As you can see with the comparisons between herbivores' and carnivores' physical makeup, they are extremely different, and it shouldn't be hard to determine which group of animals we humans belong in. We should be able to place our characteristics into one of the two categories (meat-eater, or plant-eater). However, it turns out that humans are a mixed bag of physical digestive traits.

Humans have many flat teeth that do not slide past one another (molars), and which are perfect for grinding up plants, but also have a full set of sharp canines, which, depending on your amount of overbite or underbite, do slide past one another in a slicing fashion. This diastema, or space between the canine teeth, allow for the sharper teeth to make the scissor-like motion. They aren't very long canines, which means that we do not use them as weapons for attacking or defense, but many herbivores do have very large canines, as mentioned before. The fact that we do not need our teeth for weapons means that the chewing capability is the only determinant factor.

We produce the same enzyme in our saliva that herbivores do in order to begin digestion immediately, but the stomach of a human can be extremely acidic, pH 1, which lends itself nicely to digesting meat.

It has also been noted that a particularly high intake of plant carbohydrates, which happened with the inception of farming, decreased oral health. This could mean that eating plant carbohydrates in the way we do today is not natural.

The time it takes to digest food for humans is relatively small compared with herbivores. We can get our protein in places beside plants, so we don't need to let the food sit in our stomachs for hours on end, only to regurgitate it and swallow it again to let it simmer in the stomach pools some more, just to extract the protein from grass. Rather, we can get our protein from meat (which is a great deal easier to extract protein), and all we need to take from the plants are their vitamins (also fairly easy to extract).

Although we have many characteristics of a plant-eater, the fact that we digest things so quickly makes it necessary for humans to eat meat in order to take in everything we need. According to a recent paper by an anthropologist DJ Chivers, "Humans are on the inner edge of the faunivore cluster, showing the distinctive adaptations of their guts for meat eating, or for some other rapidly digested foods, in contrast to the frugivorous apes (and monkeys)."

Something else that separates us from our plant-eating cousins is our relatively small digestive tract compared to strict herbivores, which require warehouses of storage in order to digest what they eat. Most primates are mainly fruit-eaters, but have omnivorous leanings; for instance, chimpanzees have a keen liking for ants, which tend to have a lot of protein, but do not require sharp teeth to eat. Chimps also have a taste for small animals like mice, bush pigs, and squirrels. Other primates, such as the ground-dwelling baboons, who live in the open country, seem to be particularly good at hunting small game as well as insects. These cousins of ours have been known to easily surround infant gazelles and antelopes and consume them.

One advantage humans have over many animals is our extremely adjustable jaw, or mandible. The fact that it can move back and forth and side to side makes for the potential of a good diet. No matter what the food is and regardless of our dental makeup, we can chew in such a way as to simulate a carnivore or an herbivore.

Another possible advantage that we have as humans is our eyesight. It just so happens that the most brilliantly colored foods are the ones with the most to offer with respect to vitamins and overall health value. Have you ever heard the rule of thumb that the greener the lettuce, the better it is for you? Compare the bark of a tree and the nearby orange hanging from it. To the human eye, the orange will stand out dramatically and thus will attract us more. It is not just a coincidence that the orange is better for you too. An article in <u>Health</u> magazine by Anne Underwood tells us to "Eat Our Colors." It tells of the National Cancer Institute, which has recently launched a campaign to promote foods by their bright colors called, "Savor the Spectrum." Now, we not only have a food pyramid to pay attention to, we also have a color wheel to think of. According to them, a diet of brilliantly colored red tomatoes, orange carrots, yellow lemons, green broccoli, and blue blueberries put us way ahead of man's best color-blind friend, the dog. The dog, since it is a meat-eater, focuses on motion as opposed to color in deciding what to eat. You've maybe heard that dogs are color blind. Their eyes have evolved to hunt active prey, not pick out vibrant fruits and vegetables.

How A Dynamic Physiology Helps Humans

It's all well and good that we are physically capable of most eating any type of nourishment, but does that actually benefit us, and how does it benefit us? If the availability of a particular food is limited or restricted for humans, it is reasonable to see that the ability to eat a different food puts humans at an advantage over other animals. In times of drought, common herbivores slowly die out easily because the plants that sustain them are not as readily available. But months after the plants have all died, there are still animals sticking around, stubbornly. Being able to eat those animals when there are no plants around is a big plus! It means that we humans don't starve. And when all the land animals, which have supported the humans in this hypothetical drought have been killed, there are the ocean-based animals such as fish. Before modern times, of course, the wealth of animal life in the oceans was never threatened and continued to supply fishers with endless amounts of food.

About 1.5 million to 10,000 years ago, a large animal called the mastodon roamed North America. This animal dominated in the post-dinosaur era, and it was especially well-suited for the cold ice age that existed at that time. When the major freeze subsided around 10,000 years ago, the animal, along with its cousin, the mammoth, died out. It is speculative as to why exactly they died out, but since it happened when the ice age subsided, many scientists say that the climate change affected the types of available food, thus limiting the mastodons' diet. The animals couldn't alter their diet and thus couldn't survive the dramatic climate change.

In another situation, it is quite plausible to imagine humans finding themselves in a location where there is very little fauna (or at least fauna that the we were designed to eat) and mostly just vegetation. In this case it is beneficial for humans to have teeth and a digestive system that can take in the energy of plants. When the mastodons and mammoths became extinct, one of their predators, the saber-toothed tigers lost a major component of their diet and also died out. Humans were newcomers to the area, but outlived both species because of their high ability to adapt.

The fact that humans are omnivores allows us to survive and thrive in every part of the globe, regardless of the natural disasters that may alter the food supply. Sure, it helps to have an active and large brain to help become the most dominant species on Earth, but without the ability to eat a vastly diverse diet, we may well have died out along with the mastodons or the saber-toothed tigers. A diverse menu helps us survive in an ever-changing world.

Part Three

The Cultureless Diet

(How Natural Man Would Eat)

Q: If you eat a candy bar in the forest and no one is there to see you eat it, does it have any calories?

Q: Is your idea of a balanced diet a cookie in each hand?

The human body is a tricky organism. We are designed to eat a certain way— a way that makes it easier for us as a species to exist and even thrive in adverse conditions. Yet we are also a special species, in that we are so smart and so technologically advanced, that we've gotten to the point where we don't have to work much at all to get whatever we want to eat. For those of us in developed countries, our menu is as large as our imagination. In addition to the abundance and variety of food, we humans have mastered the ability to produce hypersensitizing foods.

For example, our scientists have been able to make a substance that is 8,000 times as sweet as sugar. This means that to match the sweetness of 1 tablespoon of this super-sweetener (neotame is the name), you would need over 31 gallons of regular table sugar. Wow! Talk about a sensory explosion!

Although the super-sweeteners can be explained scientifically, there are also things the cooks in our age have been able to do without explanation. An example is the McDonald's French fry. How on earth can something so bad for us taste so good? The recent court suits, claiming that the food side dish is addictive and causes people to become fat, have shown the nature of the beast. These suits may seem outlandish from an outside perspective, but bring to light the amazing qualities of French fries: they are condensed flavor and just like the super-sweeteners, produce a sensory indulgence.

> **An Evolution Diet Essential:**
> With our scientific expertise and our seemingly weak will power, we humans are straying away from what we are naturally designed to eat.

Most people would agree that the problem isn't that these foods taste good, it's that they are bad for us as well. Additionally, we humans are designed to enjoy things that taste like French fries, and we're not designed to avoid them. We know they're bad for us and yet, they taste so good, our will power is no match.

So with our expertise, knowledge and seemingly weak will power, we humans are straying away from what we are naturally designed to eat. We are doing it, ironically because we are naturally designed to eat what we like, but how could our evolutionary ancestors have foreseen French fries? We should be able to listen to our bodies and eat what tastes good, but unfortunately, the man-made foods that taste good are doing a number on us and completely tricking our taste buds.

Some may ask, "Why do we continue to eat the way we do, knowing that it is the cause of our obesity and health problems?" How can we overlook such a detrimental aspect of our lives as our health? It is easy to simply say that we are *designed* to like the taste of doughnuts and soft drinks, and just leave it at that, but there are many reasons why we, as different cultures, eat specific things. If you are interested in why we eat specifically what we eat, we have some more exploring to do. After we have a grasp of that, we will look at how the human species would eat normally if we weren't so technologically advanced.

Cultural Influences

Besides our genes, there are many influences telling us to eat, and *what* to eat. If you are a television watcher, you might have noticed that not a series of commercials goes by without an advertisement for a fast food company or a grocery store commercial. If you are driving down the road, the chances that you see a billboard or a restaurant sign enticing you with mouthwatering images of foods are quite high.

But, if the restaurants' food wasn't appealing to us, those ads would not be very successful. So why do pictures of a hot, greasy, ten-pound hamburger look appealing? Is a human's desire for a hamburger innate? In other words, if Joe Schmoe had never before seen, tasted or smelled a hamburger, would a picture on a billboard make him want to eat it? Imagine driving down the road and looking up to a billboard with the slogan, "How long has it been since you've tasted Heaven?" And below that slogan: a picture of a large seasoned grasshopper. Doesn't that sound appealing? No? Well, it just might to some native Africans when they get hungry.

Many African groups collect locusts (grasshoppers) in the morning hours before they become active, then boil them, clean them and add a bit of salt, and voila! You have a high-protein, tasty treat. Termites and caterpillars are also popular insect foods around the world.

Beware if that sounds disgusting, we in western culture haven't removed insects from our diet completely. A food that's very popular in Western culture has been regurgitated by bees in its production, and that food, of course, is honey.

Although it may sound natural to think that certain foods

are disgusting and shouldn't be eaten, that reaction is most likely just something you've become accustomed to in the culture that you've grown up in. Food is one of the most cultural-linked things that we partake in as humans. Every culture has different styles and things they eat. Take Australia, for instance. A few years ago, when I was there, I dined at a local restaurant. When I ordered what I thought was their version of shrimp, I had no idea that the little critter would come out with its eyes bulging out and looking at me!

Australia is very close to America as far as its food goes, but this was certainly shocking. Now, can you imagine what extremely different cultures would dare to eat? I found out one day when a Chinese friend of mine took me to Chicago's Chinatown district and to a Chinese food market. My friend seemed normal to me before this trip, but when I saw her indulging in the aromas and the sights of the store, I was very skeptical of her mental state. Not to gross you out, but who can think a dried and cured pig head can look appetizing? But why stop at his head, how about a little pig's feet? It definitely gave a new meaning to the nursery rhyme *This Little Piggy*.

My favorite was the dried air bladder from a fish. My, those Chinese chefs are resourceful! Perhaps it has something to do with the fact that the country has to feed over a billion people. I can't imagine how many people we Americans could have fed with all the dried air bladders that we've thrown away in the last couple years.

But even foods that *everyone* eats are served vastly differently. Take an egg, for instance. I prefer mine scrambled, with a little salt and pepper, maybe throw some cheese on it. However, if the occasion called for it, I could find myself eating eggs poached, sunny side up, or hard boiled. These are normal ways of eating an egg to me. When I was in France, I was amused, though not necessarily appetized by seeing a sunny side up egg sitting on top of a bowl of pasta. Similar emotions came to me when I saw that the pizza I ordered came with a bright and shiny egg right in the middle. Needless to say, I ate the egg separately. Nothing could have prepared me for the whopper of egg preparations: The Chinese Thousand Year Old Egg. This masterpiece is prepared by soaking the egg in lime and brine until the egg white turns a gelatinous brown and the egg yolk turns green.

Ahhh, so that's where Dr. Seuss was when he wrote <u>Green Eggs and Ham</u>. I think I'll stick with mine scrambled.

But, perhaps *our* food isn't that appealing when you really take a look at it. What if I offered you a slimy white clump of live bacteria? Does it sound better when I add a gelatinous fruit extract? What if I packaged it, and called it yogurt; would that appeal to you? Next on the menu: a fine specimen. A cylinder of ground up jowls (the loose, fatty flesh from the lower jaw or throat), and other parts mixed in with nitrates which may cause health conditions, but keep foods very fresh! How does that sound? That may not sound very good, but when you add some mustard and relish and plop it down on a hot dog bun, it sure does taste good!

This might lead one to believe that humans can eat anything, and they pretty much can. We can derive nutrition from a vast variety of foods, so why does our culture (speaking for the Americans) like hot dogs and hamburgers, but not the Thousand Year Old Egg? Why can't I go to the concessions stand at the baseball stadium and order a dried air bladder?

Anthropologist Marvin Harris, Ph.D. at the University of Florida, who has written many books on eating says that there is an established menu in every culture and the things that aren't on our menu slowly become alien to each person growing up in that environment. He says, "When you don't eat things, you end up regarding them with disgust." There's nothing innately grotesque about a bowl of camels' eyes to eat, but since we grew up eating a bowl of cereal in the morning instead, it sounds awful.

Personal Influences

It seems that there is a period of time when we are pretty open for new foods. The first few years of life, we are usually vehemently opposed to bitter foods and generally like sweet things, but for a few years after that, we are willing to open up our palette to everything. Erik D'Amato, in an article in Psychology Today said, "By age seven or eight, children learn—or are taught—what foods to consider disgusting and in what combinations palatable or even scrumptious foods become disgusting." So, the foods that gross us out are established well before our adult lives. This happens, of course, by culture, family, and friends telling us what to eat, but also special instances unique to each individual. Experience is another important influence on our diet.

If someone has a deep aversion to chicken, it may be caused by an incident in those early years. Perhaps the first few times that person had chicken, it wasn't cooked all the way and made them sick. This would link that sickness to that particular food for their entire life, or until they decided to try el pollo loco again. I recall at one point in my childhood taking a large gulp of cola on a boat trip in the middle of summer. The cola had been sitting out in the sun and was warm. I could have sworn there was a fly in the beverage, and I took the little bug in with the drink. Needless to say, I wasn't much of a cola drinker for a while after that.

Recently, I've been able to get over my aversion to it and enjoy a tasty Vanilla Coke every once in a while, but I'm by no means the cola drinker, or the pop drinker, for that matter, that most Americans are.

First and foremost, we eat things that our culture promotes, and second, we prefer items that have a good memory associated with them. Mr. D'Amato quotes Alexandra Logue, dean of the School of Liberal Arts and Sciences at Baruch College and author of <u>The Psychology of Eating and Drinking</u>, "Liking things that are familiar also means liking things that you've eaten and that haven't made you sick."

And we are even pickier than that, due to our wealth. It baffles me to listen to some kids in today's society whine about how they won't eat a perfectly good hamburger because they don't like the pickle that was layered in between the lettuce and tomatoes and ketchup and mustard. Does this make any rational sense? I rather like the pickles, but with all those flavors running together, does it really make that big of a difference? Most likely, this is a very lucky child who doesn't know what it means to be hungry and dream of his next meal for an entire day or more.

Once, when I was eating out, I noticed a family of four sitting next to me. I overheard their conversation and noticed that one of the kids wouldn't eat his chicken fingers because they didn't look like McDonald's Chicken McNuggets. I thought, "Maybe this kid wouldn't have such a liking for the McNuggets if he knew what 'McFrankenstein' ingredients were actually in them." Either way, he was going to make a stand and not eat his chicken fingers. Eventually I think his stomach started to question his behavior and he started to pick at them, but I got the message—some of us are irrationally picky eaters.

It may seem odd that we are so picky in a situation where there is so much food, but the pickiness is most likely derived from the wealth—we can afford to be picky. This may also explain why readily available insects aren't a part of our diet and they are in parts of North Korea.

Our wealth is another reason why we don't eat what we would naturally eat. Can you imagine a group of hunter/gatherers declining to eat a buffalo they had just captured because a pickled cucumber had touched it? Not a chance!

Of course, some food may be rotten or otherwise unhealthy for us, and it may benefit us to avoid that food. In this respect, it's good that we are repulsed by some foods. A meal that might have passed for the caveman, after all, would probably make a health inspector of a local restaurant shudder.

The healthfulness of foods in our grocery aisles is certainly a great advancement in our culture, but if someone from this culture strayed from our standard of food, they might not be prepared. Imagine someone who is used to America's food standards going to Mexico for the weekend and having food that the natives eat all the time. While the Mexicans are fine eating a burrito with a little extra bacteria in it (a little Tapatió will kill it), the American would probably have adverse effects from the food—or what doctors have termed, "Montezuma's Revenge!" The unusual bacteria present in the burrito would most certainly cause unwanted indigestion, if not more violent symptoms. Thus, it is not only taste which people become accustomed to, but it is also the quality of food that people become accustomed to.

Regardless of the reasons why we eat what we eat, a disturbing fact remains. We have altered our menu so drastically that our natural selves, stripped of all culture and experience would not be able to understand what we eat or how we eat currently. If we were to rely strictly on our instincts for what to eat, there isn't much we would keep from our cultural menu.

What A Cultureless Human Would Eat

If we were to take away all of the culture-driven foods and get rid of the scientific mystery foods that have come along in the last few centuries, we would still find an enormous and tasty menu. We would still have all the yummy grains, fruit, vegetables, fish, dairy, and meats. Have you ever been to a restaurant where the menu has items with a little heart icon next to it indicating a healthy food? Our cultureless diet would have a little heart next to every item. Everything in the natural world is healthy for us to a certain extent. If that statement makes you want to say, "That's obvious!" Then you're probably not alone.

We process foods to make them last longer and taste better, but the more we process foods, the more it becomes unusable to our bodies. This includes refrigerating, cooking, and of course adding preservatives and extraneous man-made ingredients, all of which change the food's makeup from something our bodies know how to digest to something that our bodies can't use.

The goal is to eat things that are tasty as well as nutritious and usable to our bodies. To some, this may mean eating only bland foods like oats and no brown sugar. How exciting would that be? Who wants to eat just raw vegetables and grains?

You might be feeling, "If that's being healthy, then I think I'll pass." It gets less exciting for the cultureless human. He also would have to do without exotic foods. If the primitive man were in the Great Lakes region of North America, he would have to do without anything he couldn't find in his immediate vicinity: corn, wheat, apples, deer, bison, plus a good deal of vegetables. He wouldn't have the pleasure of citrus fruits, large salt-water fish, peppers, cocoa, or an endless amount of tasty wonders.

That hapless hunter/gatherer would be healthy because he would only be eating what he is designed to eat, yet probably would see eating as a chore and not the distinct pleasure that it is today. This is certainly *not* the idea that the Evolution Diet is trying to promote, yet it is important to know what we would eat and how we would eat it if we weren't being inundated with culture. From there we can apply our brilliance and creativity to eating the way we were designed, *and* making it just as pleasurable as it is currently.

> **An Evolution Diet Essential:** Prehistoric man ate all types of foods, but did so according to natural abundance. They did not have a mass quantity of sweet rolls or large plates of pasta at the ready.

To do this, I'm going to describe a hypothetical environment for our imaginary subject, let's call him Nat: a person who eats without cultural influences. First, let's give our primitive, cultureless friend, Nat, a community of people in similar natural circumstances. Next, let's assume that our community is composed of individuals that have the same physical makeup we humans have had for thousands of years, but have the culture (or lack of culture, rather) of ancient ancestors, those who may have roamed the Grate Lakes region 10,000 years ago. Based on studies by Dr. Clark Spencer Larsen of Ohio State University and others, we know that up until recently, humans on the North American continent had a nonagricultural society which gained its nutrition from foraging and, of course, hunting. We know that before agriculture took hold in North America (around 500 A.D.), the people there were predictably less sedentary and less crowded. This, in turn, led to a healthier, more active population. And it wasn't as susceptible to disease as a population densely packed into a small town or city would be. Although the cities of today allow for better and quicker health treatment with the hospital, they also aid in the spreading of sickness and disease. Luckily for us, our science has enabled us to overcome the diseases and illnesses that limited pre-modern city dwellers.

According to Larsen, the agriculturization of humans allowed for a constant supply of food, but also had drawbacks for human health. Reliance on the superfoods (e.g. rice in Asia, millet in Africa, and maize in North America) led to poor oral health, poor bodily growth, and more disease.

As mentioned in the previous part, Larsen cites an increase in these high carbohydrate foods as a cause for a shocking growth in periodontal disease around 800 A.D. in the Americas. Additionally, he notes the lack of iron in these foods as a cause of smaller bodily structures over the same time period. Finally, he states that the sedentary lifestyle of the large populations that depended on farming was "conducive to the maintenance and spread of infectious disease". These superfoods were present before agriculture sprung up, but the over-reliance on them is partly what has caused the decline in health.

So, what did prehistorical man eat if they didn't have the food pyramid to guide them? How could they have been so healthy as to make it out in the wilderness, without modern medicine or health care? Even with their highly stressful life, man lived up to 40 years of age in the Mesolithic period (10,000 B.C. to 6,000 B.C.), well beyond childbearing age.

It is probable that humans before agriculturization ate all types of food, including the superfoods like corn, but did so in a less structured, less methodical way. More importantly, they ate it according to the natural abundance. They did not have a mass quantity of sweet rolls or large plates of pasta readily available. What they did have was mass quantities of green leafy vegetables and to a lesser extent, denser vegetables like carrots and fruits like apples. Also fairly plentiful were nuts, legumes, and berries. Of course, the modern staples like grains and corn were also available.

The pre-modern man (before agriculturization) would constantly be eating these abundant natural foods to ward off their hunger. But, unlike modern humans with the ability to reach into a bag of Cracker Jacks and pull out a handful of popped corn and peanuts (complete with glazed sugar), it would take some time to get to the food that Nat, our cultureless friend would be eating. He would pick at the plant for a long period of time, slowly ingesting what nowadays we would eat in one large super-sized bite. This practice of constantly eating, but eating slowly does two things: it moderates the intake of food, thus stabilizing the intake of energy, and also keeps the eater's metabolism going. We will discuss these two characteristics in the next chapter, but keep this in mind: for the most part, Nat wants to keep eating. This is why those of us who are obese can blame their condition on their genes. We are designed to put food in our mouths constantly.

We are designed to eat mainly two types of foods—energy and protein. When Nat and his friends get enough energy from their foraging menu, they seek a more substantially nutritious food by hunting. Hunting is a non-modern person's form of exercise. To be completely healthy and as efficient as we can be as a species, we must not settle on the scant protein of nuts and plants, but rather, we must hunt (to put it into primitive terms) the extremely rich foods, which animals are. And, with the energy needs taken care of from his constant foraging of carbohydrates throughout the day, the proteins that Nat eats can go directly to body building and body regulation. I will explain the body's chemistry in the next chapter and find out why it is important to eat in this manner.

The hunter/gatherer society, which has just successfully hunted a large animal would be able to then gorge on this immediately abundant food source. And it is important that they do so to avoid the bacteria—Prehistoric man could not rely on cooking to kill the bacteria on leftovers. Although cooking is used to kill off the bacteria, which find themselves attracted to meat, humans can safely digest raw meat if eaten within a reasonable time period (one to two days). Our stomach is a powerful incinerator, which can take in just about any food or bacteria without ill effect. Even still, how we eat is important to capitalize on this trait.

When dense protein is present in the stomach, HCl is released at a faster rate and the acidity is increased in the stomach to below pH 2. This acidity enables the digestion of the protein and the killing of the bacteria. If there is a large amount of dense carbohydrates in the stomach at the same time, the pH is raised, making it more difficult for the stomach to digest the protein properly. The result is putrefaction of the meat and fermentation of the carbohydrates. This process creates a great deal of gas and makes it more difficult for the body to take in the needed nutrition. It might not be that beans are the "magical fruit," and the "more you eat them, the more you toot." Rather, it may just be that people eat beans with the wrong foods (e.g. beef) and thus, our body doesn't react kindly to them.

You can see that even though the actual foods Nat eats are fairly close to what we eat today in terms of basic components, they had a vastly different eating style than we do. Nat and his community eat one thing, like berries, for an extended amount of time and then moves on. They gain variety through time, not all at once, as in the balanced meal. They focus on one type of naturally occurring fruit or vegetable, maybe a couple at a time, and then move on to a different location and also a different plant. Then, after they hunt, they gorge themselves on meat for a number of days. They do not have the food pyramidal diet of every food group in each meal; in fact, the idea of a meal is completely lost with the Nat. While they do get all of their vitamins and minerals, they do so in a less uniform manner.

This style of spacing out their intake of different foods optimizes their body's ability to focus on certain things and change the reaction to what's in their stomachs. This style of eating extracts the most nutrition from the food they take in as well as keeps their metabolism going on a fairly consistent path, one that their body is designed for.

Part Four
The Body's Chemistry
(What Our Body Does With the Food We Feed It)

"The toughest part of a diet isn't watching what you eat. It's watching what other people eat."
-Dieter

Q: If you split a can of diet cola with one calorie into two glasses, which glass gets the calorie?

      There are four different types of things the body needs in order to have a completely healthy life: Building Materials, Life Process Facilitators, Energy, and Water.
      The Building Materials we need are amino acids, which are used to build proteins. Without these materials, we would be barely anything but water and fat. The Life Process Facilitators are the vitamins and minerals, which alone do many things such as protect against free radicals, help you digest certain things like calcium, and help in every basic life function, like burning energy.

There can be no replacement for vitamins or minerals or amino acids, but there is nothing more important to our health than water. Water makes up over 60% of our entire body weight and is impossible to live without. A human can live weeks without any food energy, but only a couple days without taking in any water. We're lucky that water can be found in almost everything we eat. One doesn't have to drink 8 glasses of water a day to stay healthy because it is in the fruits and vegetables and to a lesser extent meats, and breads that we eat all the time.

The main choice that we have in our diets is what form of energy we eat. Since we can get energy in four very distinct ways, there has been much debate over what the best way to attain our energy is, as anyone who has been on an extremely low carb diet can attest. The four forms of edible energy are carbohydrates, proteins, fats, and alcohols. All have unique attributes that make them beneficial or deleterious and, as with most things we can ingest, there is a limit to how much one should be eating of each. I will discuss each energy type in exciting detail and explain the pros and cons for each one.

Carbohydrate Is Not A Four Letter Word

With recent diets on the market such as the Atkins plan, many people have gained an extreme aversion to the friendly little molecules of carbon and water (hydrogen and oxygen = hydrate). Some people have gone so far as to ban the energy type from their diet, entirely. Some people have taken measures so drastic to limit their carb intake that it seems like just eating less altogether would be easier and less painful than adhering to such a strict gimmicky diet. It appears our culture has gotten a little out of hand: commercials promoting a beer with 1 gram of carbs fewer than a competitor's; orders at a restaurant like, "Could I have the burger meal deal, no bun, no tomato, hold the fries, but could I get a little cup of the grease you fry them in?" endless supermarket trips with constant pursuing of the ingredients panels looking for the zero carb food that tastes good; people having nightmares of little carb monsters chasing after them.

The Evolution Diet is here to stop the madness! Carbohydrates are not the end of the world and, in fact, they are quite necessary for optimal health. Diets like the Zone and Atkins push the unending benefits of protein as an energy source and blame all health problems on carbohydrates. Those methods of eating may help you lose weight also, but they will be contrary to what your body is designed for and cause a significant amount of stress on the inner workings of one's body.

What's In A Carb?

Carbohydrate is the general term for an extremely versatile type of molecule. There are two main types of carbohydrates that we digest: simple sugars and complex carbohydrates. There is a very important difference between the two because the body treats them extremely differently. Although they are both made of the same basic components, they are composed in very different ways. The basic chemical formula for a carbohydrate looks like this: $C_6H_{12}O_6$. This is the simplest form of a carbohydrate called glucose.

Glucose is the preferred energy source used by all the cells in our bodies. When we intake other types of sugars, they are broken down into glucose so that the cells can use it. Glucose is so simple, that there is absolutely NO digestion needed to make the substance useable by our cells. If you were to sip a yummy glass of fresh glucose juice, the glucose molecules would flow directly from your digestive tract and into your bloodstream, hence another name for glucose: blood sugar.

The fact that it can enter our bloodstream so quickly without any middleman is a benefit, in that it can give us a boost of energy when we need it, but can also be a hazard. If you need that instant kick, a frothy glucose beverage is just what the doctor ordered, but if you're not in any need of energy, this boost might make you irritable, tense, or annoyed. Our bodies have their way of regulating this spike in energy, but the effects are still potent, especially when one ingests pure glucose (or simple sugars).

Tips On Energy Sources

- A calorie is the energy it takes to heat 1 gram of water by 1 degree Celsius.

- What people call a calorie everyday is actually a kilocalorie, or 1000 calories defined above.

- A gram of carbohydrate has 4 calories, a gram of protein has 4 calories, and a gram of fat contains 9 calories.

- 3,500 calories is equivalent to 1 pound of fat.

- Although most nutrition labels cite a 2,000 calorie diet, the actual recommended intake for an average active person is 2,500 calories per day.

- It takes the human body different amounts of time to get to the energy contained within different food types.

You might say, "But I've never ordered a frothy glucose shake." Perhaps you haven't ordered it by name, but every time you open a soda can you're drinking that glucose straight. You can find glucose in honey, grape juice, and corn, which produces a form of glucose called cornstarch. Other fruits have a similar molecule in them called fructose, which has the same chemical makeup as glucose, but the atoms are in slightly different places. Galactose is another one-celled sugar, or monosaccharide, but is only found naturally connected with glucose. Fructose and galactose can also take rides through our bloodstream because they are so simple. More complex molecules need a little bit of work before the body can use them directly.

Interestingly enough, glucose is about half as sweet as table sugar, which is a disaccharide that contains a glucose molecule and a fructose molecule. Disaccharides (meaning contains two monosaccharide molecules) are just a bit more complicated than the single molecule sugars, but are broken down very easily in our digestive tract, as well. Common disaccharides are sucrose (table sugar), lactose (the sugar in milk), and maltose (the sugar in, you guessed it, malt).

Glucose Molecule ($C_6H_{12}O_6$)

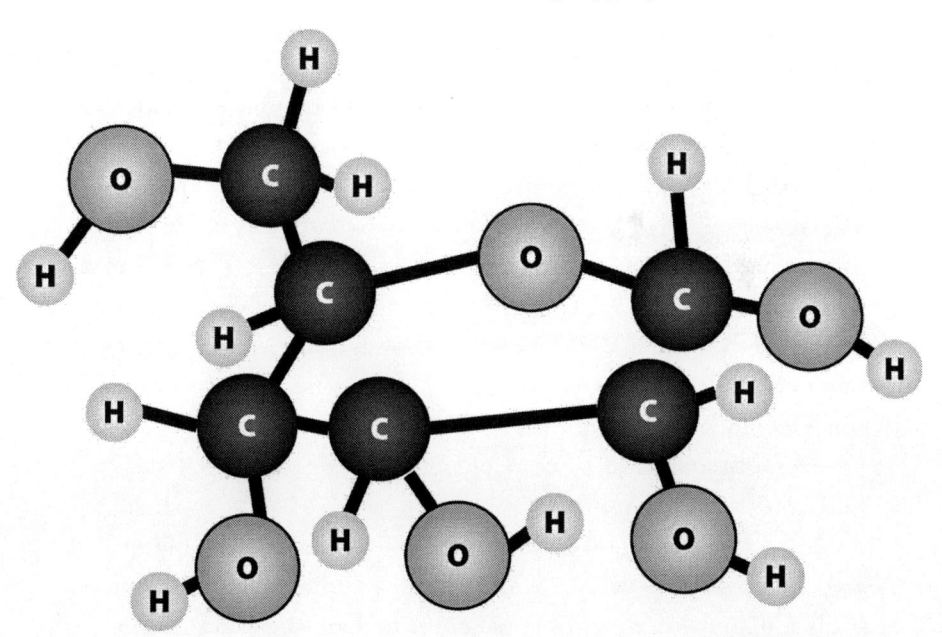

Source: HOW STUFF WORKS

Sugar definitely gets around, and has many pseudonyms. If you want a laugh sometime, look on the ingredients of a candy or a candy bar and count the number of ingredients which are really different names for the same thing: sugar. A Snicker's bar lists that same ingredient (sugar) five times as different pseudonyms. Pop Tarts list that same ingredient nine times! Manufacturers can disguise the name sugar as any of the following: corn syrup, dextrose, lactose, galactose, fructose, galatactose, glucose, high-fructose corn syrup (HFCS), honey, invert sugar, levulose, molasses, or sucrose.

These all taste sweet, which is an immediate indication of its potency. These sugars are ready to get the body going, and fast! If you eat a good amount of a simple sugar, you should feel the effects immediately.

You should feel more awake, more alert, and you should have more strength and energy. This is the immediate result, though it's not sustained. All of us have, at some point, experienced the lull after a sugar high. Perhaps you've had one too many soda pops or you've eaten candy for an hour straight, and you've been wired and bouncing off walls for the last half hour, when all of the sudden, you start to come down. This is your body catching up with you. The sugar high that you just had was a result of mass quantities of glucose being released into the bloodstream — much more than was needed for normal operation. The average human body needs about two teaspoons of glucose to do what it needs to do at any given time and a lot of that comes from the more complex energy sources that you've been digesting for the last few hours. When you take in foods with sugar as the number one ingredient, you're most likely taking in three to four times as much glucose as you need. If you drink a soda pop, you're putting in three tablespoons of sugar, or four and a half times the needed amount, in your body.

There are a few organs that are involved in controlling your blood sugar level, your hypothalamus and your pituitary glands in your brain, and the pancreas in your abdomen. There are little peanut-like formations of cells spread out on the pancreas called the Islets of Langerhans. Instead of picking on these little guys because of the funny name, you should know that these guys produce one of the most important hormones in our bodies: insulin.

Insulin controls the amount of blood sugar in your blood, and if your body is only used to a little glucose coming in at a time, as is the case for most people, it's going to take a while for those little peanuts to crank out the needed insulin to regulate the blood sugar. Insulin feeds the glucose to the cells (sugar high), and when the cells are all full, the same hormone, insulin, brings all the excess glucose in the blood to the liver to convert it to a complex carbohydrate (and you feel the sugar low). If you took in too much sugar for even that process to handle, the excess glucose is converted into fat. There is an appropriate amount of sugar the body should intake and we will discuss that later.

With such an amazing amount of stress caused by glucose, it's hard to imagine that it's good for you at all, but it is extremely important. While there are three monosaccharides that can flow through the bloodstream, glucose is the only energy source that the brain can use. Maintaining your glucose level is important, not only for energy, but also mental wellbeing. Fortunately, you can eat complex carbohydrates to receive the glucose you need and you can avoid the drastic sugar highs and lows that simple sugars cause.

What Does Too Much Sugar Do To Us?

We know that our body tries to maintain a constant blood sugar level and the ups and downs of that level contribute to a high level of stress by our internal organs. When this stress becomes too high for the body to handle, bad things can happen. Diabetes Type II is one of those bad things. When there is an excess caloric intake (eating too much) with a deficient caloric expenditure (exercise, metabolism), the body fights against itself. First, it starts to ignore that ever-important enzyme insulin. Then, the body stops producing it all together, and when the body's natural infrastructure that deals with maintaining blood sugar levels is tampered with or damaged, one has to maintain those levels manually. This is why diabetes patients must inject themselves with insulin on a regular basis. If you aren't so keen on needles, it might be a good idea to take it easy on the sugar.

This diabetic self-maintenance of blood sugar levels can be done safely and effectively, but often involves a dramatic shift in one's lifestyle and behavior. If a diabetic doesn't moderate their blood sugar, the results can be blindness, and a lower life expectancy. There are other less critical symptoms; webMD lists some interesting symptoms as the following: Feeling dizzy, tingling, blurred or distorted vision or seeing flashes of light; seeing large, floating red or black spots; or seeing large areas that look like floating hair, cotton fibers, or spider webs. It's quite possible that if you were at an Allman Brothers' concert in the '70s, you might have been sharing these symptoms. As odd as these symptoms may seem, diabetes is a serious illness and must be treated as such.

When something as important as insulin is not being made by your body, that means that your body is not working for you any more. The rise in diabetes in Western culture can be attributed to people's diets not conforming to the way we were designed to eat. The Evolution Diet aids your body and helps its natural processes to regulate insulin and to alleviate the stress caused by unnatural eating habits.

One of the key factors in preventing diabetes is eating for your lifestyle. One should only eat a lot of sugar if they are expending a lot of energy. That makes perfect sense, right: you should take in what you expend. The only reason you need to overload your system with a mouthful of sugar is when you're running or kayaking, or playing dodge ball.

You may notice that if you do eat a candy bar or drink a glass of orange juice, and you're not exercising, you may feel energetic, wired, or even anxious or irritable. These are natural reactions to a bulk of sugar entering your bloodstream. It is your body telling you to use that energy and go exercise.

The Yale Guide to Children's Nutrition explains that the body's reaction to high sugar foods is cause for some adverse effects if we aren't eating for any purpose other than energy. If one eats an excess of sugar and doesn't use it, there could be problems:

> ...when a child eats a sweet food, such as a candy bar or a can of soda, the glucose level of the blood rises rapidly. In response, the pancreas secretes a large amount of insulin to keep blood glucose levels from rising too high. This large insulin response in turn tends to make the blood sugar fall to levels that are too low 3 to 5 hours after the candy bar or can of soda has been consumed. This tendency of blood glucose levels to fall may then lead to an adrenaline surge, which in turn can cause nervousness and irritability... The same roller-coaster ride of glucose and hormone levels is not experienced after eating complex carbohydrates or after eating a balanced meal because the digestion and absorption processes are much slower.

The last part of this is extremely important, "The same roller-coaster ride of glucose and hormone levels is *not* experienced after eating complex carbohydrates..." (e.g. breads, white potatoes, vegetables, and high-fiber foods). Although these foods have very high amounts of carbohydrates, the amount of sugar is relatively low so it is more difficult to digest and get to the energy. It takes an extremely more complex process to get to the basic glucose molecules in broccoli or French bread than a soda pop.

When you intake high-sugar foods your body takes in glucose at a rate of 30 calories per minute, while a complex carbohydrate gives you just 2 calories per minute. That's a whopping 15 times the ingestion rate. If you were to eat the same amount of calories in garlic bread as in a glass of grape juice, you would notice no sugar spike with the bread and a dramatic spike in blood sugar levels with the juice.

Something you may have heard a great deal about recently is the glycemic index (GI) of a particular food. It is the rate that the given food increases one's blood sugar. This index is extremely questionable in its clinical legitimacy, but the concept is good. Some foods affect your body with increased blood sugar more than others. Within the category of fruits, apples have a low GI (38), while dates have a high GI (103). The low glycemic foods are great for constant eating throughout the day in low quantities and the high glycemic foods are suitable only for before and during exercise.

Note that while the glycemic index may be telling of the potency of each particular food, it is also important to factor in another trendy term: the glycemic load. While the glycemic index is measured by judging the equal weights of foods (50 grams of carbohydrate from apples compared with 50 grams of carbohydrate from dates to arrive at the figures listed above), it would be a lot more difficult to eat fifty grams of apples, since they are relatively light. This is important when you see something like the glycemic index of carrots (131). When compared with pasta, which has a GI of 71, carrots seem very bad for you, but one would have to eat a pound and a half of carrots to eat the 50 grams necessary to get to that 131 GI.

Another thing to keep in mind when you look at the glycemic index of foods is the control substance used to achieve the GI. There are two common comparisons: glucose at GI 100, and a slice of white bread at GI 100. These two different controls give extremely different variations of GI, although they are always proportional. A baked potato has a glycemic index of 85 compared to pure glucose, but a whopping 121 compared to white bread. Brown rice is GI 55 compared to glucose and GI 79 compared to white bread. If you were to compare the wrong figures of brown rice and a baked potato, you might think that they are very similar (85 to 79), but in reality their glycemic effect is vastly different, according to these studies.

There are some obvious flaws with the index, however. If you compare breakfast cereals, for instance, you will find that sugarless Corn Flakes has a relatively high GI of 80, while a sugary cousin, Frosted Flakes has a GI of 50. Pretzels are also pretty high with a GI of 83, but a snickers bar is a healthy 41 GI. If this makes you scratch your head about the glycemic index, you're not alone. The American Diabetes Association has not endorsed the index, citing high amounts of doubt in its clinical utility. The ADA says that priority should be given to amount, rather than the source of carbohydrate.

In general, if you want to determine how a particular food is going to affect your blood sugar, listen to your taste buds. A food that is dense and sugary is going to spike your blood sugar—no matter what you mix it with.

We Are Made of Protein

That title is almost correct. We're actually only 20% protein, another 60% water, and the rest is minerals (e.g. calcium in your bones). A person without protein however, would look a lot like one of the scary skeleton pirates from *Pirates of the Caribbean*. A healthy person has a wealth of protein. An interesting thing about protein is that we can pretty much run on protein alone. Protein is so nutritious that it contains all we need to make energy, promote growth, and aid in digestion of minerals. The question is then, why do we eat anything else?

Humans can do just about anything with amino acids, including use them for energy, but it's extremely stressful to use amino acids for anything but building blocks. In fact, for the body to use proteins as energy, the body must imitate its reaction to a high amount of stress. During high amounts of stress, fat is mobilized from storage (converted to sugars), blood sugar increases, blood pressure increases, minerals are drawn from the blood and proteins from the thymus and the lymph glands are turned into sugars immediately.

When there is little availability of carbohydrates, the body turns to protein metabolism for energy. The first step is the breakdown of proteins into smaller amino acids and sending these molecules into the blood stream, increasing blood pressure. While amino acid content in the blood is high, the body releases two opposing hormones, insulin and glucagon. Insulin lowers the blood sugar level, while glucagon raises it. These two hormones are usually released at different times to regulate blood sugar, but during protein metabolism, they are both needed to ensure the process. This is okay in people who aren't diabetic, but is considerably more stressful than if one's diet included carbohydrates.

The second step of protein metabolism is the break down of the amino acids into what are basically a carbohydrate structure and a nitrogen component. This nitrogen unit is great when paired with a carbon unit, but is pretty useless alone, and in fact, it is dangerous at certain levels. The nitrogen unit (usually ammonia) is removed from the blood stream through the kidneys.

> **An Evolution Diet Essential:**
> If there are ample amounts of carbohydrates in your diet, you can use those for energy, and use proteins for what they are best at: cell building. If you have no carbohydrates in your system, your body will use protein for energy.

The near-carbohydrate unit, called a carbon skeleton, can then be used for energy. If this process seems like a lot of stress to get a couple of calories of energy, you're right. If there was an ample amount of carbohydrates in the diet, the person would be able to use that for energy and use proteins for what it is best at: cell building. In addition, an appropriate level of carbohydrates will reduce blood pressure and the poisonous nitrogen content in the body, reducing unnecessary stress on the liver and kidneys.

Having stated the danger of consuming solely proteins, it is necessary to note that the body can't survive on just carbohydrates. The body needs protein and most peoples' diets today are deficient in protein.

Humans need what are called amino acids, which are found in proteins. The body distinguishes these amino acids into two categories: essential and nonessential. We can make the nonessential amino acids from other things in our bodies, but we

The Body's Chemistry | 49

cannot create the essential amino acids ourselves, so we must get them from the food we take in.

The Recommended Daily Allowance of protein is .36 grams per pound of body weight. A person who weighs 160 pounds would need to consume 57.6 grams of protein a day. A small can of tuna has 33 grams, so you can see that it doesn't take much to achieve the recommended amount. When you exercise, however, your body requires more protein to rebuild the muscle tissue you've just damaged and build more. Conversely if one doesn't exercise, one doesn't need as much protein.

Regardless of the amount of protein in one's diet, it is vital for the intake of the important building blocks that you eat them separately from mass amounts of carbohydrates. In Dr. Rush's paper, "Applying Medical Anthropology: Gut Morphology, Cultural Eating Habits, Digestive Failure, and Ill Health" he describes how large amounts of dense carbohydrates interfere with the digestion of protein. In this passage he mentions the body's ability to digest the two different types of food differently:

> When protein enters the stomach, the hormone gastrin is released which causes the release of HCl, lowering the pH level to 2. This is necessary to begin the process of denaturing the protein and cleaving peptide bonds. However, when dense carbohydrates (fats are less of a problem) are added to the meal, they interfere with the activity of HCl and other *acid* enzymes for properly breaking down the protein. Further, the carbohydrates raise the pH level of the stomach contents and this signals the release of more HCl. However, the carbohydrates, once again, raise the pH level, and the process goes on and on leading to a burning sensation (gastritis), gas and bloating, and uncomfortable fullness. The protein, then, is *not* being digested.

50 | The Evolution Diet

He also attributes common problems like heartburn and acid reflux "disease" to the poorly conceived diets that combine carbohydrates and proteins into a supposedly magical USDA balanced meal. The human's reaction to different foods and the specialized way in which we digest them is most likely due to the humans' natural eating habits. Natural Man would pick at a food (most likely a high-fiber carbohydrate) in a certain area and then hunt an animal and eat their fill of that. And, they wouldn't eat a potato found near the beast they just hunted- the potatoes will be there long after the animal prey will. In other words, they wouldn't be eating protein with fruits and vegetables.

Amino Acid Molecule ($C_3H_4O_2NH_3$)
Amino Acids are 1 part of a protein molecule.

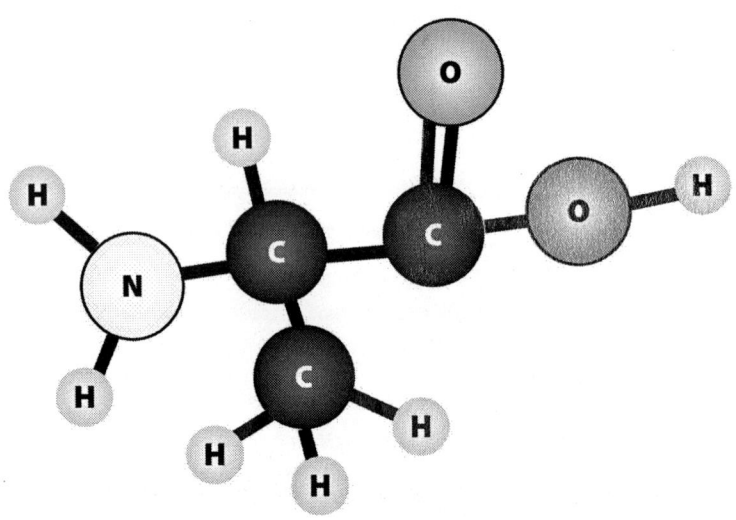

Source: HOW STUFF WORKS

Since this hunting usually took place during broad daylight, it is assumed that the gorging of the animal occurred in the evening leading to a sleep. Although many specialists ask their patients not to eat a large meal before sleeping, it is actually a natural behavior, especially if it's a large protein meal. Many high-protein foods actually contribute to good sleep. Anyone who has eaten too much turkey during Thanksgiving will attest to the sleep-conducive powers of the turkey amino acid, tryptophan.

And, it's not just turkey that has this snooze stuff. Cheese, milk, tofu, seafood, beef, poultry, eggs, and nuts also have a good amount of tryptophan.

With the notable exception of bananas, very few high sugar foods have a lot of tryptophan. Our bodies are designed to eat the food listed above in high quantities before rest, while the high sugar/carbohydrate foods should be limited before sleep. The Evolution Diet asks you to eat your proteins at the end of the day, preferably after exercise, and before sleep in order to help you sleep.

Tryptophan takes about an hour after consumption to reach the brain, so this might be taken into account when planning your eating schedule. Also, the earlier you eat, the sooner you will be hungry the next morning. If you have trouble sleeping, it may be caused by hunger. The larger the meal and the later it is, the more it stifles your digestion and prevents you from suffering from hunger throughout the night.

With Friends Like Fats, Who Needs Enemies?

Just like protein, we need fats to lead a healthy life, so in a way, fats are our friends. There are two major functions (besides energy) that fat has: vitamin absorption and bodily support.

Although the most commonly known roll of fat is to store energy so that we may go days without food, another integral roll for the food is the digestion of vitamins. There are thirteen vitamins essential for humans and four of those require fat to be present to be used by the body. These fat-soluble vitamins protect against things like night blindness, rickets, anemia, and poor blood clotting.

Another vital role fat has is on the cellular level. Just like certain amino acids from proteins, we need certain fatty acids from fats that we can't create ourselves. These essential fatty acids support the cardiovascular, reproductive, immune, and nervous systems. They come in two forms that you may hear in advertisements: Omega-3 and Omega-6 fatty acids. Along with the nonessential fatty acid Omega-9, these are the good fats.

You can find these essential fatty acids in foods as diverse as flax seeds, salmon, peppermint leaves, soybeans, and shrimp.

It is important to note that, with regard to energy, fats are fairly easy to burn. Since we store all of our excess energy as fats, though, our bodies see fat as excess energy and without added exercise, the fat will remain as fat and not be turned into energy.

There are two main types of fats, which represent what people call the good fats and the bad fats: unsaturated and saturated. Saturated fats are those that are solid at room temperature and these are the bad fats with very little benefits. These fats usually come from animal sources and include lard. Unsaturated fats are the more beneficial types and the essential fatty acids are in this category. These fats are liquid at room temperature and come from plant sources, most commonly olives, peanuts, and soybeans.

Some oils are not 100% unsaturated, though. Check the nutritional information and ingredients to get the content of the oils before you buy them. If you have some oils with saturated fat content, you can separate the two by placing the oil in the refrigerator. After a couple hours, the saturated fats will separate and become solid.

There is one type of man-made fat that everyone should be particularly aware of and should make a concerted effort to avoid. That fat is hydrogenated or partially-hydrogenated oil. As mentioned before, oil is a type of unsaturated fat, which can be healthy in moderation. Oil from vegetables such as olive oil, which is a mono-unsaturated fat, can help reduce blood cholesterol levels and help reduce the risk of coronary disease. However, food production companies started altering natural oils in the beginning of the 20th century and what they created was extremely unhealthy.

By heating natural oils in the presence of a metal catalyst and hydrogen, liquid oils turn solid. The benefit of this was its ability to replace more costly natural solid fats like lard. The production and use of these trans fats increased until the 1960s and health benefits were even attributed to them. Unfortunately, they are extremely bad for us and have a uniquely adverse affect on blood lipid levels and lead to coronary disease.

Many countries in Europe have planned the banning of all

Fat Molecule ($(CH_2)_2CH_3(COOH)_3$)
Fat is also known as a triglyceride.

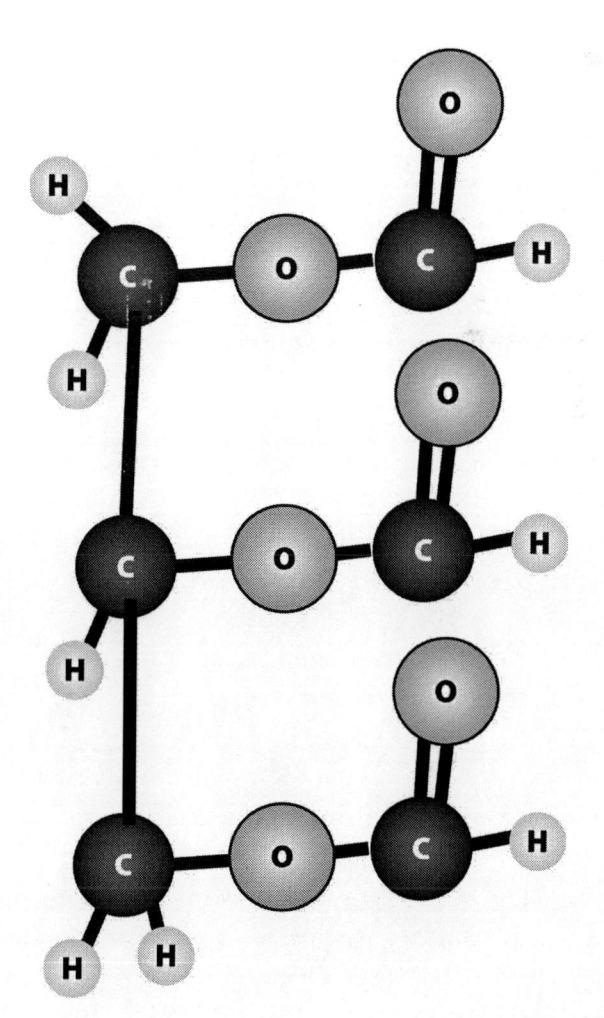

Source: HOW STUFF WORKS

trans fats in food, and the US Food and Drug Administration has seen enough evidence to require food producers to list the fats on the nutrition labels. Until then, you can identify unhealthy foods by looking for "hydrogenated" or "partially-hydrogenated oil" in the ingredients. Avoid these as much as possible.

Part Five
The Evolution Diet
(Now We're Ready to Get Started)

"It's something most of us do religiously: We eat what we want and pray we don't gain weight."
- Anonymous

"For some, dieting is a *weigh* of life."
-Anonymous

In reading the last few sections in this book, you may be finding yourself questioning your own diet. You may be thinking that the food you used to eat is nothing near what your body is asking for. You might be suddenly aware that the food you used to consider healthy is now known to be detrimental to your health. If you are questioning your current diet—that is first step to eating the way you were designed to eat.

"But what I eat tastes so good! Maybe I can't eat the way I was designed to eat." It's understandable if you find the thought of a new diet daunting, but you can do it and the rewards are well worth the effort. If you push yourself for a couple days, eventually you will regain the natural rhythms of your body and you will start to crave the natural method of eating. Soon, you won't be able to eat any other way because you will enjoy the way you feel so much.

Although the actual science behind The Evolution Diet is complex and somewhat confusing, the simple principles are easy (after all, Natural Man followed it without the benefit of science). I will go over the basic fundamentals of the diet, then go into an extensive day-to-day plan for the average person. I will follow with some things to consider while you are *eating to evolve* so that you may maximize your potential health.

The Fundamentals

With our standard of living today, there is no excuse for being unhealthy, whether that means underweight, overweight, or simply without proper nutrition. The main factor preventing the majority of people from attaining perfect health is will power. They can't fight the urge to eat the highly calorie-saturated foods, or they can't find the drive to exercise at least every other day. The Evolution Diet can solve both of these problems by allowing dieters to eat what they want (for the most part), but to eat those things at different times of the day and in different amounts than they're used to. Simply altering their eating schedule will give them energy when they need it and, more often than not, an added drive to exercise when their bodies tell them to.

If you are trying to do any of the things listed in this book like lose weight, get more energy, sleep better, get rid of daytime lulls in energy, become more alert, or just become healthy, all you need to do is follow four principles. It may sound too good to be true, but it's not rocket science.

Once you begin to get back to the way you were designed to eat, it will be easier for you to work even harder on your health. All you need to do is get the ball rolling, so to speak, and you will be rewarded, almost instantly.

The first step is already taken care of: you've acknowledged that you'd like to change some things in your life. You wouldn't have bought this book otherwise. Now all you need to do is the next four things and you'll be on your way.

There are four main principles of The Evolution Diet:

1. Listen to your body.
2. Appropriate your diet.
3. Avoid intake of Artificially Extreme Foods (AEFs).
4. Exercise and sleep when your body tells you to.

These principles, though seemingly obvious and simple, are the key to living a perfectly healthy life and need a thorough explanation. We will get to exercise and sleep in a later section, but we will discuss the first three now.

Listen to Your Body

One of the most common mistakes people make when they are in bad shape is that they don't listen to their body. They usually find themselves eating a bag of potato chips out of boredom or nervous habit, when they should be eating ONLY when they're hungry. If people followed this principle alone, they would lose weight and/or feel dramatically better.

The fantastic thing about this principle is that you don't need any crazy gadget to follow it; you have an automatic meal timer and calorie counter built in with you. Hunger pangs are your cue to start looking for more food. The trick is to decipher between actual physical hunger pangs and other things that compel us to eat like boredom, stress, or habits such as the mechanical reaction to the lunch bell. This seems obvious, but the key is to eat only when your body is telling you, not for psychological reasons.

Physical hunger pangs are the direct indication that your stomach is shrinking as a step in digestion. When your stomach does this, your metabolism begins to slow down, which means you begin to lose energy, store fat, and your endocrine system starts to kick in causing unneeded stress. To avoid slowing your metabolism you must satisfy your hunger with a small amount of natural low sugar, high fiber food.

That means that people who like to eat constantly are in luck. The Evolution Diet allows for constant snacking throughout the day. This is because you will not be eating large 1500-calorie meals every 4 hours; you will be eating small quantities of moderately difficult foods to digest. Like we went over in Part 4, natural foods are more difficult to digest than typical fast food. One can pick at food constantly, all day, if they so chose, as long as it isn't the super-artificial foods, like French fries or doughnuts.

The types of food that are perfect for this constant eating in small quantities are low in sugar and high in fiber, or what we will call LoS Hi-Fi foods, and other carbohydrates with a moderate amount of fat and protein. But, before you bite into that slab of cardboard next to you, read what tasty snack foods are perfect for this period of the day:

It is important to note that a common serving size for

LoS Hi-Fi (Low Sugar, High Fiber) Foods

- Mixed nuts
- Crackers and salsa
- Fresh broccoli with fat-free ranch
- French bread with olive oil and vinegar
- Triscuits with cheese
- Multigrain Cheerios with milk
- Blueberries
- Toast and butter
- Bagel with cream cheese
- Lightly buttered popcorn
- Carrots and celery
- Salted edamame
- Pita with hummus
- Salad greens with low fat dressing

most of these would be far too much to eat in a matter of minutes. You will notice when you eat just a couple bites, you almost immediately thereafter lose the sense of hunger. If you listen to your body, it will tell you to leave the rest of the snack for later. Eat these foods in small, regulated portions so that you don't get to the point when you feel stuffed, or even full. For instance, say you eat and orange and a small bowl of cereal for breakfast and the first time you're hungry after that is at 10 am. Eat 2 crackers with cheese. In about twenty minutes you may feel a little hungry again—have three bites of broccoli with fat free ranch and so on until you're ready for exercise or dinner.

> **Case Study: Bettie**
> Age: 36 Goal: Weight loss
>
> Bettie started the Evolution Diet after 10 years and 80 pounds of weight gain. She had three surgeries to help maintain her weight. She confessed to lack of motivation and, "needless to say, I am not happy with myself."
>
> She picked up the Evolution Diet quickly and took immediately to the snacking portion of it. "I really enjoy just munching on something during work, and although I can't just eat any time, I can whenever I get a hunger pain. I love the types of food I eat at my desk: [no candy] snack mix, and cucumber and tomato salad with fat free Italian dressing. The amazing thing is, I'm probably eating more than I ever have, or at least I feel like it, and I've already lost 15 pounds!"

Remember, there is a happy medium between the hunger pangs you feel and the full feeling you have after eating too rapidly. It is important to maintain this happy medium if you want to eat how your body is designed to eat. This will take some discipline at first, but once you get the hang of it, you will not want to eat any other way.

Appropriate Your Diet

The part that people have the most trouble with in their diet is eating specific foods when their body needs them and only when it needs them. You were designed to eat certain foods at certain times because those foods provide your body with timely benefits. There are basically three types of good foods: complex snacks or LoS Hi-Fi foods, high energy foods, and high protein foods. LoS Hi-Fi foods provide your body with sustained energy throughout the day; high energy foods give your body a boost before and during exercise; and high protein foods rebuild your body and prepare you for sleep. They all have a specific time to be eaten according to your activity level. But there are a number of factors in modern culture working against this appropriation. Cultural superfoods, fast food, and, believe it or not, the balanced meal are just a couple of the agents working against your health. All of these go against what your body is designed to consume.

You may be eating perfectly healthy foods, but there is a great chance that you are not achieving perfect health if you do not appropriate certain food for certain activities. For example, eating too much sugar before sleep would make you restless at night and tired the next day.

Without appropriating your diet you could be overweight, nervous, tense, easily stressed, a horrible sleeper, and so on. These could all be due to the body not getting what it needs with regard to energy and nutrients at the right time.

As Omberto, an Evolution Dieter, likes to put it, "There is food for work, food for play, and food for the rest of the day." This is the essence of appropriating your diet.

Good foods must be eaten at the right time to truly be good. For example, an orange is a very nutritious food that provides vitamins that help bolster our immune systems and prevent diseases like scurvy. We can easily employ the energy we get from an orange, and the moderate amount of fiber it contains regulates our digestive tracts. So, an orange should be considered a healthy food.

But, if someone ate five oranges in an hour, it would *not* be healthy. The easily digested sugars in an orange would make the orange-happy person shoot around like the Tasmanian Devil while the high acidity in the orange may cause an imbalance of pH in the stomach. Also possible is an overabundance of vitamin C. All vitamins become toxic at certain levels, and while humans can take in and use a super-high amount of vitamin C (RDA of vitamin C is 60 mg, while the toxicity level is somewhere around 25,000 mg), it *is* possible to have too much of it. With all this being said, it is easy to see how eating so-called healthy foods does not always contribute to health. There is such a thing as "too much of a good thing." Moderation is the key to eating the way we would naturally eat things.

In the same way that eating too much of a healthy food is bad for you, so is eating certain foods at the wrong time. Both dietary flaws give you something your body doesn't know what to do with.

Conversely, it is *beneficial* to eat certain foods at the right time. You may have heard of good foods to eat before you sleep like a warm glass of milk or cottage cheese. Just as there are good foods to have before sleep, there are good foods that you should eat during the day, before exercise, and when you are tired.

Complex carbohydrates are perfect throughout the day because they offer a constant flow of energy, enough to allow the body to perform optimally without spiking blood sugar. Sugars are good before and during exercise to ensure a sustained, high-energy output. They are also handy when you need a little pick-me-up or when you're feeling tired, but can't afford to sleep. When you are not dependent on sugar and not constantly eating sweets (like many of us do), a high-sugar food will kick up your energy before you can say, "Maltodextrose."

Of course, the most valuable thing we put in our body, water, should be consumed consistently throughout the day. Especially good times to drink it, though, are before meals and after you wake up. If you are trying to lose weight, water is a great way to trick your body into thinking that it is fuller than it is. When you mix a tall glass of water with your regular high protein dinner, you tend to eat less since you feel more of a bulge.

Protein is perfect after exercise and before rest and sleep. Since exercise damages your tissue (most notably your muscles), your body asks for the rebuilding materials after you are done working out. When you eat protein after exercise, your body knows exactly what to do with it and doesn't start detrimental protein metabolism to turn it into energy and ammonia, as explained in the previous part. If your body gets too much protein, which is what happens when you eat it at the wrong time, the body stores it as fat or gets rid of it all together, creating additional toxins in the body.

High Protein Meals

- Chicken burrito with cheese with black beans with a chipotle salsa
- Grilled turkey salad with low-fat dressing
- Crab-stuffed salmon steaks on a bed of spinach
- Filet mignon steak with cheese artichoke side
- Grilled tuna and bean salad
- Southwestern omelet with tomato, avocado, and honey-glazed ham
- Caesar salad with grilled chicken
- Hamburger lettuce wraps with roasted asparagus
- Barbequed chicken with green beans
- Ham and cheese crêpe with broccoli and cauliflower
- Roasted salmon with macadamia cilantro crust and squash
- Cajun flavored crab legs and lobster tail with whipped cauliflower

Protein also makes for a good pre-sleep meal because it usually contains the essential amino acid tryptophan, which brings the energy level down and aids sleep. Protein is digested slower than an equivalent amount of complex carbohydrates.

Also, when you eat a large amount, no matter what the food type, you will be tired immediately after because more energy will be required for heavier digestion.

With The Evolution Diet, one can eat to their heart's content around dinnertime, as long as one is eating high-protein foods. Around 70% of your dinner, in weight, should be protein. A method of determining this is found in Part Nine. The body's metabolism is running constantly at an even pace, gaining energy throughout the day until you eat a large dinner of fish or cheese or egg or soy. This change in the digestive process is healthy and coincides perfectly with your natural sleep cycles. It should be noted that the size of a high protein dinner should be proportional to the amount of exercise done before.

Let's review. To eat what and how you would naturally eat involves snacking on foods that are low in sugar and high in fiber with a little protein throughout the day to sustain a high and level amount of energy. It is acceptable to eat natural high-energy foods before and during exercise, but only if your goal isn't to lose weight. A couple hours after exercise or a few hours before sleep, you should fill yourself with a 70% protein meal and very little sugar (5% at most). Your high-protein meal should be big enough to tide you over through sleep, but if you're hungry after dinner, you should have a high-protein dessert like cottage cheese with a few slices of a peach.

Avoid Artificially Extreme Foods

When you awake, the cycle starts over with moderate intake of complex carbohydrates and a little bit of protein. Some people may need a little extra boost in the morning. If that's the case for you, an orange or a small glass of orange juice will be able to do the job that would require 3 or 4 cups of espresso before the Evolution Diet. Although caffeine can be found naturally in many foods, coffee is considered one of the Artificially Extreme Foods because it is easy to

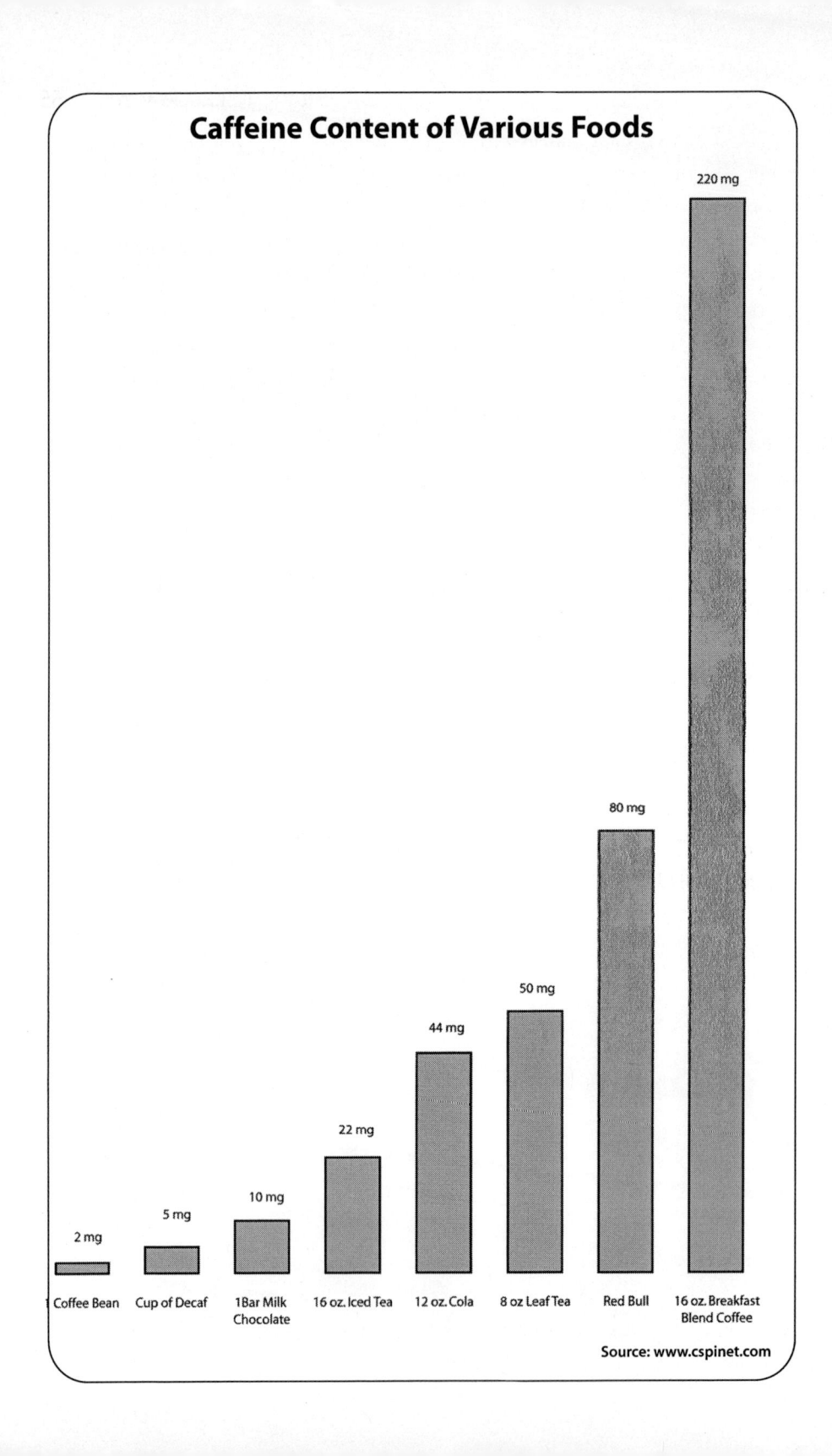

Caffeine Content of Various Foods

Item	Caffeine
Coffee Bean	2 mg
Cup of Decaf	5 mg
1 Bar Milk Chocolate	10 mg
16 oz. Iced Tea	22 mg
12 oz. Cola	44 mg
8 oz Leaf Tea	50 mg
Red Bull	80 mg
16 oz. Breakfast Blend Coffee	220 mg

Source: www.cspinet.com

Case Study: Cindy
Age: 25 Goal: Better sleep, Weight loss

It took Cindy an emergency in the family to alert her to health. Although she has always been relatively healthy, she wanted to eat better. "As a result of my father's stroke (he is ok, in a residential rehab program) my mother and I have decided to try to become healthier together. I have joined a gym and she has started going on morning walks with our dog. The problem is eating. We both have weight to lose (she has much more than I do) and want to eat healthier food, but don't really know where to start or what to change.

"I would love to lose some weight (I just graduated from college and gained a lot of weight while enjoying my senior year), maybe 10 pounds or about that, and get healthy. I just started my first real job but it is not causing too much stress in my life, but I am more stressed than I used to be. And I NEVER sleep well anymore without the help of sleeping pills (which I try not to take more than twice a week and only when necessary, I don't want to become addicted)."

She has been taking off the pounds since she started (about 8 lbs. at the time of the writing) and she's found the high-protein meal in the evening the key to better sleep. "Since I began eating almost all protein at night after my exercising, I've gotten really tired about 3 hours after the meal. I didn't know a change in diet could do so much to my physical state. The sleep has been unbelievable! I wake up and don't feel like I've just been tossing and turning all night. I feel energetic and spunky in the morning. It's fantastic- I don't think I'll ever change the way I eat now."

achieve an excess intake of it with the modern serving portions.

One coffee bean, found in nature has about 2 mg of caffeine. If someone were to eat coffee beans in nature they would probably get bored after about 15, maybe 20, and they would get a nice little kick from caffeine soon after (caffeine takes about an hour to take effect). A person sitting down to a tiny cup of espresso is taking in the equivalent of 50 coffee beans! Of course, one serving doesn't quite suffice for those of us who order the medium grande triple shot, iced latte con panna with a little lemon twist. That's has an amazing 330 mg of caffeine! Yikes!

Although caffeine has some immediate benefits to health like increased awareness, increased breathing, and appetite suppression, a diet with caffeine as a major staple is extremely unhealthy. Becoming dependent on the drug will decrease your stress and exercise tolerance in addition to causing irregular heart patterns, increased blood pressure, and aggravation of digestive tract problems like ulcers. If you're someone who, "Can't live

Case Study: Tom
Age: 25 Goal: Higher Energy

"I'm a healthy guy, for the most part," Tommy explained, "but I can't get rid of these lulls in energy that I get throughout the day. Sometimes it gets so bad, I fall asleep at my desk at the insurance company." That's definitely something to be concerned with. When Tommy explained his old diet, it was clear as to why he was experiencing his lulls in energy. He usually had a cup of Bella Vista F.W. Tres Rios® Costa Rica coffee with two sugars from Starbucks in the morning, and maybe a glazed scone if he was feeling hungry. Usually he wasn't, so he was providing a nice little boost of energy for himself—first from the sugar, then from the caffeine. But when that boost was done, he might have been hungry, which would without a few cups of coffee a day," that should be your first indication that the dependence has started. Your body was not designed to handle such a stimulant constantly.

And the effects can be lasting, if not permanent. An article in National Geographic noted an interesting scientific experiment about brain activity in heavy caffeine drinkers versus non-caffeine users. It showed that the brain activity of a coffee drinker and a non-coffee drink was relatively the same, but only when the coffee drinkers had caffeine in their system. When the coffee drinker didn't have any caffeine or when the non-drinker did, the differences were dramatic. In essence, the body likes a certain level of brain activity and if you are constantly feeding yourself a stimulant, the body will compensate for that and return to the normal level of activity.

The psychoactive drug, caffeine, is a nice pick-me-up when you really need it (e.g. when you're driving late at night), but when you become dependent on it, caffeine is only holding you

---

have lowered his blood sugar, and he would have no sustainable energy source in his system except for a few grams of complex carbohydrates from the scone. Since he always had his coffee and sugar in the morning, his body had come to depend on that boost. When he became tired a couple hours after, he rightly assessed that the caffeine was wearing off, but he would just drink another cup.

Once he replaced the coffee and scone with a couple slices of buttered toast and an orange, he felt energetic throughout the morning. There were no more lulls caused by the absence of caffeine. He got his energy from the long-term source of complex carbohydrates. This energy source leveled out the spikes and lulls into a constant supply.

back.
     Coffee is just one of the Artificially Extreme Foods (AEFs) which I have mentioned a couple times in this book. There are a number of AEFs that make more sense to avoid, such as fried foods, foods with partially-hydrogenated fats, and super-sweet foods like soda pop. The major problem with these foods or additives is that they are more than our body is designed to handle, which is due to the fact that we've made them stronger than they can be found in nature. While we can handle just about anything for a short period of time, extended periods of

> ### Case Study: D'Shauwna
> Age: 31 Goal: Motivation, Higher Energy
>
> **Mrs. White came to the Evolution Diet as a slightly overweight woman who was lacking motivation and didn't really have much energy. "I am not lazy—just have a hard time eating 3 meals a day and my metabolism has stopped, I think. I know that exercise is important to me, but whenever I try to get motivated, I can't imagine anything worse." D'Shauwna was used to eating a large mixed bag of protein and carbohydrates for lunch. After work she expected to feel like exercising. Quite the opposite, D'Shauwna was telling her body that everything was fine in the world of nutrition. In essence, exercise is the component of our modern lives that is linked to hunting and gathering. Since our dieter had stuffed herself in the middle of the day, that made her feel content without "hunting" for substantial food.**
>
> **We got D'Shauwna on a routine of eating small amounts of complex carbohydrates throughout the day, and a little sugary boost right before she was going to the gym. Viola, she had, "More energy than [she] ever has had," before exercising. She was shocked, but getting rid of a giant meal in the middle of the day and filling the gaps with small food made her prepared, even excited for exercise.**

intake of such foods will lead to serious problems like heart disease, high blood pressure, diabetes, or cancer. It is important to avoid these foods whenever possible.

Some AEFs are natural originally, but are so concentrated or distorted that they are harmful to our bodies. Oranges are found in nature, but to get an 8-ounce glass of orange juice, one must squeeze 8 to 10 oranges. If one ate 8 to 10 oranges, they would doubtless be quite full with all the fibrous healthy bits in the rest of the orange. Orange juice is an AEF because it is a source of such highly concentrated sugar that it is not natural even though its derivative is natural. The same goes for fried foods.

> ### Some Healthy High-Energy Foods
>
> - Oranges
> - V-8 Splash
> - Carrots
> - Yams with sugar glaze
> - Grapes
> - Frosted Flakes
> - Carrot cake
> - Strawberries
> - Granola bar
> - Raisins
> - Trail mix with dried fruit and candy
> - Peanut butter and Jelly
> - Banana pudding with 'Nilla Wafers
> - Orange sorbet
> - Bananas

Although saturated fat is found naturally in animals, the concentrated amount that is used to deep fry foods is impossible to find in nature.

Although the Evolution Diet is a fantastic way of taking what you normally eat and rearranging it to optimize your body's mechanical processes, there are certain foods which you must give up to attain better health. Although there are some instances when you would need to replenish your blood sugar with something like soda pop, but this only occurs during extreme physical output (exercising for more than an hour). Even then, it is recommended that you drink something with other benefits than just energy or sugar. Orange and grape juices are high-energy drinks but have other benefits like vitamin C (100% of your recommended daily allowance in a small 8 ounce glass). Different drinks can be deceiving also: a can of Coke has nearly twice as many grams of sugar as the same amount of Gatorade, a beverage that promotes its energetic attributes.

> **An Evolution Diet Essential:**
> Humans naturally want a bit of food in their stomachs at all times. But you should replace the Snickers bar with highly fibrous foods to maintain the naturalness of keeping something in your stomach at all times.

You may be asking, "Well, if I can't eat anything as sweet as a doughnut or as filling as a pound of chili cheese fries, doesn't that take all the fun away from eating?" The answer is NO. When you begin to eat foods the way we were designed, you'll begin to appreciate more subtle flavors in food. In the Evolution Diet you will re-sensitize your taste buds and enjoy a wider range of foods.

I was reminded of the desensitization factor recently on a mountain in Arizona. One day we were heading out to snowboard and ski, and before we hit the slopes, we wanted to get a good amount of sugar into us so that we wouldn't get tired throughout the day. I had a bowl of instant oatmeal with a lot of sugars, a Danish, and a couple of glasses of orange/cranberry juice. I then had a bagel that tasted pretty bland, so I put butter and jam on it. I took an additional bagel with me to eat later that day. After a couple runs down the mountain, including about 15 wipeouts, I began to get hungry. I pulled out the bagel and my brother and I ate a couple bites. To our surprise, the same bagel that had tasted bland a few hours before, tasted extremely sweet on the mountain. At breakfast, I hadn't noticed any flavor in the bagel, but a few hours later it tasted almost like candy. The intense sugars we ate in the morning distracted us from tasting the flavor in the bagel. But the forthcoming exercise had warranted the intake of some AEFs.

So an argument can be made that some Artificially Extreme Foods are appropriate in certain situations, like extreme exercise. However, it's important to use common sense; a fried Twinkie, for instance, is not one of those appropriate AEFs. This goes for fat as well as sugar. We need a moderate level of fat in our diet to digest some of the vitamins we eat, but excess fats and, to a lesser extent, excess sugars go directly to storage fat for the next time we're in a famine or something devastating like that. Although real famines are not laughing matters, it can safely be said that most of us in Western culture will not have to go weeks without food, so we don't need that excess fat.

Being able to store fat is a great way for us to live through times without food, but it is a very stressful process and it harms us when we take it to the extreme. It is an unfortunate statistic that obese people live an average of 7.1 years less than people with an ideal weight, while overweight people live slightly longer than obese people. In a shocking report by the University of Illinois at Chicago, it is estimated that life expectancy for Americans will actually decrease for the first time in 2005. The main reason for this is the increase in obesity. One third of the US is obese and an additional one third are overweight.

The single-most important factor in the overweight epidemic is the abundance of these Artificially Extreme Foods. Studies have shown that the average American diet increased calorie intake by 10% from the mid 1970s to the mid 1980s. They didn't see an increase in serving size (however shocking that may seem); they saw an increase in the caloric density of foods. When you add that higher caloric density in foods with the enormous sized portions we eat today, it's no wonder that the majority of Americans are overweight.

The bright side of this is that it's never too late for you to correct this problem. You can start with the next bite you eat. The way to do this is eat the way we were designed to eat, not the way the television or our schedules tell us to eat.

Humans naturally want a bit of food in their stomachs at all times. In addition, as we've noted, they can handle large quantities (of protein) when needed. But when you replace the low calorie, high fiber foods found in nature with high density, jam-packed foods like a Butterfinger candy bar, there is a problem: you will be hungry in a shorter while than if you had eaten a couple stalks of broccoli, but you will have taken in 10 times the amount of calories.

There are certain techniques out there that focus solely on certain aspects of the Evolution Diet. The Pritikin Principle is to eat foods that have lower calorie per pound ratios. It is not too hard to see how the more processed foods are, the more calorically dense and extreme they are. Natural corn off the stalk is a sweet 490 calories per pound, while tortilla chips at the friendly neighborhood Mexican restaurant are 2,450 calories per pound!

Hunger is an urge telling us to fill up our stomach, and it can be sufficed by something as simple as water. Water is easily digested, however, and a glass of water won't hold back your hunger very long. Water, though, is a great supplement to snacks. A couple tasty little multigrain crackers and a glass of water will make you just as satisfied as if you were to eat a Snickers bar. Snickers has easily digested sugars and does not satisfy, contrary to the way its advertisers may want to portray the candy. Water is also an important supplement when you're eating dried foods like the fruit in a bag of trail mix. Since the fruit is dehydrated it will take you a lot more to fill yourself than if you were eating fresh fruit. Dried foods usually have much higher caloric density than their hydrated counterparts. It doesn't help that dried fruits usually have added sugar.

Part Six
Sample Diet
(What The Evolution Diet Looks Like)

Day 1

Breakfast:
1 orange
Half a banana muffin
Small glass of skim milk

Daytime (eaten over a period of 9 hours):
Triscuit crackers (about 12)
Water
Half a banana muffin
4 Strawberries

Exercise:
20 minute walk

Dinner:
Small tossed greens with low-calorie dressing
Salmon steak with teriyaki sauce and a cilantro pesto spread
Whipped cauliflower with butter
Water

Day 2

Breakfast:
Small bowl of bran cereal with low-fat vanilla flavored soy milk
Small glass of Carb Countdown Orange Juice

Daytime (eaten over a period of 9 hours):
1 Temale
Water
5 saltine crackers
Half a banana

Exercise:
3 mile jog

40 pushups
100 sit-ups

Dinner:
10 oz steak fillet with salt and pepper seasoning
Steamed broccoli with cheese
Diet caffeine-free cola
Water
1 chocolate candy for dessert

Day 3

Breakfast:
2 Low-fat toaster waffles with low calorie syrup
Tall glass of 1/2 calorie orange juice

Daytime (eaten over a period of 9 hours):
Banana
Fresh broccoli with zero fat ranch dressing
Water

Exercise:
None

Dinner:
Small plate of pasta with meat sauce and 2 large meat balls
Glass of red wine

Day 4

Breakfast:
2 oranges
1 Hawai'ian bread roll
Small glass of skim milk

Daytime (eaten over a period of 9 hours):

2 oz of blueberries
10 Triscuit crackers with cilantro/avocado hummus
Diet lemon/lime soda
Water

Exercise:
6 mile jog

Dinner:
3 slices of meatloaf with red wine marinara sauce
8 stalks of asparagus
2 oz of cottage cheese with seasoning

Day 5

Breakfast:
Small bowl of corn cereal with skim milk
Small glass of apple juice

Daytime (eaten over a period of 9 hours):
Half a bag of popcorn
Small Greek salad
1 16 oz V-8 Splash Light

Exercise:
20 minute walk

Dinner:
6" meatball sandwich
4 mozzarella cheesesticks
1 glass of red wine

Day 6

Breakfast:
2 oranges

2 slices of whole wheat toast with butter
Large glass of 2% milk

Daytime (eaten over a period of 9 hours):
Triscuit crackers (about 12)
Water
10 carrots bites

Exercise:
40 minute walk

Dinner:
Large baked chicken and cheese burrito with Tapatío sauce
Black beans
Water

Day 7

Breakfast:
Small bowl of Cheerios with low-fat vanilla flavored soy milk
Small glass of orange juice

Daytime (eaten over a period of 9 hours):
Triscuit crackers (about 12)
15 baked potato chips with salsa
Fresh broccoli with zero fat ranch dressing
Water

Exercise:
3 mile jog

Dinner:
Small mixed greens salad with zero fat Italian dressing
Cajun-flavored Alaskan crab legs
Shrimp cocktail
2 small lobster tails
Half a slice of key lime pie

Day 8

Breakfast:
Small bowl of corn cereal with skim milk
Small glass of apple juice

Daytime (eaten over a period of 9 hours):
5 Triscuit crackers
Small Greek salad
Diet caffeine-free cola

Exercise:
40 minute walk

Dinner:
Large Caesar salad
2 ham and cheese crêpes with cream sauce

Day 9

Breakfast:
Small bowl of corn cereal with 2% milk
Small glass of apple juice

Daytime (eaten over a period of 9 hours):
Half a bag of Popcorn
Water

Exercise:
3 mile jog
40 pushups
100 sit-ups

Dinner:
2 crab cakes

1 large swordfish steak with capers and lemon sauce
Mixed steamed vegetables with seasoning
2 glasses of wine

Day 10

Breakfast:
2 low-fat toaster waffles with low calorie syrup
Tall glass of Carb Countdown pineapple/orange juice

Daytime (eaten over a period of 9 hours):
Banana
Fresh broccoli with zero fat ranch dressing
Water

Exercise:
None

Dinner:
2 pieces of thin-crust meat-lovers pizza
6 fried zucchini pieces
Water

Day 11

Breakfast:
Small bowl of bran cereal with skim milk
Small glass of Carb Countdown Orange Juice

Daytime (eaten over a period of 9 hours):
Fresh broccoli with zero fat ranch dressing
30 small pretzels
Water
1 cup of hot tea

Exercise:

None

Dinner:
Small plate of wheat pasta in a butter sauce
Glass of red wine

Day 12

Breakfast:
2 oranges
2 slices of whole wheat toast with butter

Daytime (eaten over a period of 9 hours):
Triscuit crackers (about 12)
Water
12 carrots

Exercise:
40 minute walk

Dinner:
Large buffalo chicken wrap with cheese, lettuce and tomato
Tomato, cucumber, feta cheese salad with low-calorie Italian dressing
Water

Day 13

Breakfast:
Small bowl of oatmeal with brown sugar and milk
Small glass of grape juice

Daytime (eaten over a period of 9 hours):
15 baked potato chips with salsa
5 leafs of fresh broccoli with zero fat ranch dressing
Water

Exercise:
3 mile jog

Dinner:
Small mixed greens salad with zero fat Italian dressing
Large crab-stuffed salmon steak
Steamed broccoli with cheddar cheese
1 glass of red wine
Water

Day 14

Breakfast:
Small bowl of corn cereal with 2% milk
Small glass of grape juice

Daytime (eaten over a period of 9 hours):
Half a bag of popcorn
2 slices of French bread
Water

Exercise:
3 mile jog
40 pushups
100 sit-ups

Dinner:
Large burrito with egg, cheese, bacon, sausage
Mixed steamed vegetables with seasoning
Diet A&W root beer

Day 15

Breakfast:

Small bowl of oatmeal with brown sugar and 2% milk
Small glass of orange juice

Daytime (eaten over a period of 9 hours):
Mixed vegetables with zero-fat ranch dressing
10 saltine crackers
Water

Exercise:
20 minute walk

Dinner:
4 pieces of baked chicken
Green beans
7 chunks of pepper jack cheese
Banana for dessert

Part Seven

Other Factors
(What Else Can Play A Part In Your Health)

"An old friend of mine said she lost 28 pounds just by skipping every day. She skipped dessert, she skipped the candy bar after lunch, she skipped the pancakes..."
- Anonymous

There are a number of factors outside of one's diet that affects their weight and wellbeing. I will address them in the following section. In matters concerning weight loss and energy, diet is the number one factor, but there are other things that work with and against your diet to affect your health.

Basal Metabolism

Everyone needs a different amount of calories in their diet to live. The basic functions of life (breathing, pumping blood, producing body heat) take up the largest portion of the average person's energy output. These basic functions are called basal metabolism. The basal metabolic rate, or BMR, is the amount of energy those functions consume while at rest in room temperature (68 degrees Fahrenheit).

There are many factors that play into your BMR at any given time—how tall you are, how much you weigh, what kind of exercise you're used to, and your age among other factors. There are other important factors like amount of muscle mass, but they are very difficult to determine without sophisticated equipment. The most accurate way to determine your BMR is to measure the exchange of oxygen and carbon dioxide through your lungs. This shows what you're taking in to fuel your cells and what you're throwing away. Without that equipment, you can determine your BMR with this equation called the Harris-Benedict formula:

Adult male BMR: 66 + (6.3 x body weight in lbs.) + (12.9 x height in inches) - (6.8 x age in years)

Adult female BMR: 655 + (4.3 x weight in lbs.) + (4.7 x height in inches) - (4.7 x age in years)

Determining your BMR is a great way to gauge how much you should be eating. If you don't exercise, you should only be eating the calories represented by your BMR. Calories burned from exercise (see chart in Part 8) can be added to your BMR to determine how many calories you burn in a day.

The generally accepted average for caloric intake is 2000, which is the standard on the Recommended Daily Allowance. But you may find that you do not need to be eating that much, or you may realize you need to be eating more to compensate for your high expenditures.

Basal metabolism is extremely important to your weight because it is by far the highest calorie burner working for you. The Evolution Diet is designed to keep your metabolism going at a steady pace, and thus burn more calories than you may be doing right now. When you eat the LoS Hi-Fi foods continuously in small amounts when you're hungry, you are keeping your metabolism up, and burning more calories.

Additionally, The Evolution Diet involves eating foods that

> **Tips to increase your BMR**
>
> • Turn down the heat or air conditioning. Your body expends more calories in cold or hot temperatures.
>
> • Don't binge and purge. Chronic dieters with low calorie diets lower their BMR below that of their average intake.
>
> • Choose your stress wisely. Short-term stress increases your BMR, long-term stress decreases it.
>
> • Get more muscle. Having more muscle mass increases your BMR, even when you're not using your muscles.
>
> • Fidget. Believe it or not, people who have high levels of "spontaneous physical activity" have a significantly higher BMR, on average.
>
> • Exercise. When you work your cardiovascular and muscle systems, your body must "heal" them afterwards, thus increasing your BMR for up to 12 hours.
>
> • Breathe freely. The more you hinder your breathing, the more you stifle your basal metabolism.

take more energy to digest, also increasing the daily calorie expenditure. Foods like fiber and complex carbohydrates are more difficult to digest than sugars, and that's why we avoid candy.

Exercise When Your Body Tells You To

Exercise may be one of the most important aspects to health. Although one can maintain an ideal weight without exercise, perfect health is impossible without at least a moderate amount of physical activity; the more the better. Exercise has been promoted early and often throughout history and it's no wonder: people who exercise live longer, on average, than do their couch potato counterparts. Additionally, the life they do lead is dramatically more enjoyable.

As we discussed earlier, it is vital to have a steady habit of exercise, however, the Evolution Diet will help no matter what the participant's physical activity is like. The reason for this is that the Evolution Diet restricts what a person can eat if all they do is rest. Unappealing as it may seem, without exercise, people should only eat the LoS Hi-Fi foods throughout the day—often, but in small portions. They should never gorge themselves on protein because, in nature, that would only happen after exercise (which is hunting to Natural Man). Without exercise, only small quantities of protein should be eaten and it should be eaten in the snacking manner of the LoS Hi-Fi foods.

> **An Evolution Diet Essential:**
> Exercising allows a more dynamic diet, complete with large protein dinners and sugars in addition to the LoS Hi-Fi foods.

In addition, sugars, though tasty would not be necessary if one did not exercise. Sugars tend to spike blood sugar (as discussed before) and, if not used just turn to fat. It would be easy to utilize the energy spike if you were prepared to exercise, but if you were sitting at your desk and got an energy boost, it would naturally be wasted and all of that excess sugar would go straight to the spare tire. In the meantime, it might make you irritable or tense.

So, exercising allows for a more dynamic diet, complete with large protein dinner, and sugars in addition to the LoS Hi-Fi foods.

The Evolution Diet provides a couple of guidelines for exercising that will help maximize the benefits of your work out.

1) Exercise when you are hungry or have a small amount of food in your stomach, not when you are full. When your body begins to work its muscles, your body automatically switches its focus from the digestive system to the muscles. Blood that would have gone to the stomach to aid in digestion goes instead to the quadriceps or triceps. This switch, involving vasoconstriction and vasodilatation of different body tissues, slows the nonessential bodily activities, and during exercise this means the digestive tract. The problem with this is that the stomach does not receive the blood it is used to getting for the process of digestion and cannot function properly, commonly producing the side effect of cramping.

Thus, you should follow the adage that, "One shouldn't go into the pool or ocean right after eating a big meal." This only applies to when you are exercising in water because cramping increases your risk of drowning. If water has a relaxing effect on you, it may be better for you and your digestion to wade in the pool for a while.

If you are used to eating highly sugary foods, then being hungry before exercising may reduce your energy and motivation to exercise. If you are constantly on a sugar high, being hungry may make you hypoglycemic and weak feeling. However, if you maintain a steady intake of LoS Hi-Fi foods before exercise, your body will not stress out without immediate sugar and you should have sustained energy to exercise.

2) To lose weight, exercise when you are tired. This may seem odd, but it really works! Your body becomes tired for different reasons, one of which is low blood sugar. When you have low blood sugar and you push your body in the form of exercise, the body pulls the energy from stored sources, like fat.

You can also apply this to long-term exercising as well. After you've been exercising for a couple minutes, your body starts what's called aerobic exercise. This form of physical activity uses oxygen to break down the glucose that's stored throughout your body in places like the muscles, the liver, fatty acids, and in extreme situations like starvation, glucose can be derived from protein in this process. This extremely complex process ends with the muscle cells producing energy (through the wonder molecule ATP).

3) If you get a boost of energy while you are stationary at work or at the home, use it. Get up and walk to the water cooler; go walk up and down a couple flights of stairs or walk around the block; clench and unclench your fists to get the blood flowing. If you don't mind looking a little silly, do some stretches in your office or do leg lifts behind your desk. Your body will reward you with a relaxed, yet not tired, feeling afterward. If you use the sugars that you eat immediately when they come in, you will not stress your endocrine system, as described earlier. Also, you will not retain all of the excess, unused energy as fat.

The Origin of Exercise

Natural Man did not exercise in the sense that we now know it. The people who lived before agriculture did not go to their local "gym" and lift stones every day after gathering food and painting on caves, but they were physically fit. Their form of exercise was walking from camp to camp as they followed their food sources of plants and animals.

They were continuously moving around to get fresh picks of nuts, berries, and plants that were the staple of their diets. Then, when they had enough energy from their foraging, they would set off on major hunting expeditions. Running for miles or sprinting, then attacking their prey (buffalo, deer, wooly mammoths, etc.). This physical activity was a part of the lifestyle of all natural people, not just the "man of the cave."

If the natural people were near water, they would take spears out to the lake or the ocean and, in a physically exhaustive procedure, they would spear their meals.

The reward for the physical activity, for them, was mass quantities of meat.

Today, we emulate the act of hunting by exercising. In our modern world, we should only eat mass quantities of meat when we deserve it. That is, we should only eat meat after physical activity or exercise.

The Importance of Exercise

I was out one evening for dinner with a few friends and one of the girls with us decided to go outside to have a smoke. While she was gone I noticed that she had barely touched her meal and it appeared as though she was done. She was fairly thin, possibly because her smoking habit suppressed her appetite and thus she didn't eat as much as the average American. However, she certainly was not healthy.

Although many people are thin or skinny without exercise (some because they smoke), one cannot be truly healthy without at least a moderate amount of physical activity. This is an important aspect of life. The Evolution Diet can benefit you even if you're not exercising, but it does require you to limit your intake of some foods.

During exercise, the human body requires a high amount of sugars to burn. In addition, exercise tears down muscles and works the systems of the body like the cardiovascular and respiratory systems. This tearing down process requires protein to rebuild the bodily mechanics in a healthy way.

It only stands to reason that without exercise, one doesn't need as much sugar or as much protein. If one's body could talk to them during a stretch of not exercising, it would tell them that it doesn't need so much energy or building blocks. Contrary to the 3 square meal approach, it is not always healthy to eat so much food when the eater is not exercising.

Every type of food serves its own special purpose, and it just so happens that a lot of the food we eat is only required when or before we exercise. This is why exercise is such an important part of not only the Evolution Diet, but also your general health. Organizing one's diet in the stages of the Evolution Diet (snacking on carbs throughout the day and eating a large protein meal at night) will help them, regardless of physical activity. But eating appropriately, according to the amount of exercise one does, is extremely vital for optimal health.

Breathing and Sleep

Breathing is vital to good health and, if you are trying to lose weight, it is even more important to focus on it. Breathing increases the good components in your blood (oxygen) and decreases the bad (carbon dioxide), but it also determines how fast you burn calories. When someone measures your basal metabolic rate (explained earlier), they determine how much oxygen and carbon dioxide are exchanged during breathing while you're at rest. When we exercise, we breathe more, which is a product of and an indication that we are burning more calories.

Breathing is involuntary, meaning that we breathe without thinking about it, but we can also control our breathing and in extreme cases, we can restrict our breathing physically or subconsciously. Apnea is a condition in which the person stops breathing for 10 seconds or longer, 5 to 50 times an hour. It usually happens during sleep, but can happen while awake. There are three types of sleep apnea: obstructive sleep apnea, central sleep apnea, and mixed sleep apnea. The causes may include obstructive facial features, or enlarged tissues in the nose or throat, but stem mainly from factors that you can alter yourself.

If you think that "holding your breath every once in a while" is not that dangerous, you may want to reconsider. Sleep apnea contributes to coronary artery disease and high blood pressure. In addition, sufferers of sleep apnea may experience lower alertness in their daily lives, memory problems, personality

These Hinder Your Regular Breathing Patterns:

- Drinking alcohol affects the region of the brain that controls breathing.

- Obesity affects 70% of the people who suffer from sleep apnea.

- Prescription drugs for allergies, depression or anxiety also increase the risk for sleep apnea.

- Stressful situations usually force people to limit their breathing—it becomes rapid, but shallow and doesn't provide the oxygen or other benefits of deep breathing.

- Bad posture may hinder the body's ability to open up the lungs during breathing.

- Anger focuses your body's attention on the subject of your anger, not on your biorhythms—so be happy.

changes, lower desire for sex, anxiety, and depression. Obviously, sleep apnea also decreases the quality of sleep, which in itself is important.

The quality of sleep in general has an important effect on weight loss. David Rapoport, MD, associate professor and director of the Sleep Medicine Program at the New York University School of Medicine in New York City says that sleep effects one's appetite, "One of the more interesting ideas that has been smoldering and is now gaining momentum is the appreciation of the fact that sleep and sleep disruption do remarkable things to the body — including possibly influencing our weight."

The reason for this is sleep's effects on the hormones leptin and ghrelin. When you don't have a good night's sleep, the body drives up the levels of ghrelin, which stimulates your appetite. It also drives down the other side of the balance, leptin, which creates fat cells from excess blood sugar and signals to the brain that you are full.

When you have a bad night's sleep, in the case of sleep apnea, you are breathing less and thus burning fewer calories and you are increasing your appetite for the next day. The result is weight gain, usually. "I've had about thirty patients who, when successfully treated for their sleep apnea were able to lose weight—possibly because they had more energy, so they were more active and they just ate less," says Michael Breus, PhD, a faculty member of the Atlanta School of Sleep Medicine and director of The Sleep Disorders Centers of Southeastern Lung Care in Atlanta.

Unfortunately, the converse is also true: if one doesn't treat sleep apnea, they may become overweight or obese, which, in turn, would contribute to their sleep apnea further. The vicious cycle stops by learning to sleep well, then eating better.

Hypoapnea, or slowed breathing, is also a problem that causes similar, though less extreme results as apnea. Hypoapnea can easily occur as a result of stress, so take a deep breath, and read on!

Stress

Our emotions are inextricably linked to our weight. Our state of mind and the emotions it produces directly triggers certain hormones in our body to be activated. Those hormones shooting around our bodies are so powerful, they can affect many things, most notably illness, physical strength, memory, disease, appetite and weight loss.

Stress is a dramatic emotion that we are bound to have throughout our lives. The interesting thing about stress is that it is good for us in the short term, but extremely bad for us in the long term. Our bodies were designed to naturally deal with fear and stress on a regular basis in order to cope with, say, bears that are trying to eat us, for instance. But when we translate that fear into long-term anxiety, the body's reactions aren't life saving, they're life threatening.

Immediate stress caused by a barking dog produces the hormone adrenaline in our bodies. This hormone tends to speed up our regular metabolic rate, increase breathing and heart rate, and for a very short time promote weight loss. However, long-term stress (like an anxiety disorder) produces the hormone cortisol, which stores fat (usually around the abdominal region). When you compliment cortisol with an unregulated cultural diet, you will see massive weight gain.

The first goal for a stressful person should be to identify the sources of stress for them. This may come from all types of areas: the job, irritating people, disorganization, etc.

The solution is not the many pharmaceuticals on the market. In fact, those pharmaceuticals may contribute to other problems like the aforementioned sleep apnea. The solution is to determine what is stressing you out and limit it. It could be your job, your family, or too much food. Although changing jobs may seem like a drastic step just to lose a few pounds, it may be the only way you will truly cure your stress. In turn, you will live a dramatically more fulfilling life.

Better yet, learn to relax in situations when your life is not at risk. For the vast majority of people in Western culture, this happens to be all the time. When you are focusing on your health and on what your body is telling you, you will begin to notice all the overreactions you may be experiencing that are caused by stress. You may notice that your breathing is not free flowing or relaxed. You may be stopping your breathing all together. You may be so tense that muscles all over your body are tight.

One way to reduce stress is to be an optimist. Remember to keep positive and look for the good out of every situation. If something has already happened in your life, there's no sense in worrying about it. Calmly figuring out what to do is the only way that you can overcome your obstacles.

If you don't learn to relax when you're not physically at risk, your weight will suffer. This should be enough motivation to get you to relax about the situations in your life.

Part Eight
What You Get In Return
(What Are the Benefits?)

A woman walked up to a really old man rocking in a chair on his porch. "I couldn't help noticing how happy you look," she said. "What's your secret for a long, happy life?"

"I smoke three packs of cigarettes a day," he said. "I also drink a case of whiskey a week, eat fatty foods, and never exercise."

"That's amazing," the woman said. "How old are you?"

"Twenty-six," he said.

There are an endless array of conditions and symptoms that modern people have that can be totally wiped out if we would just eat how we were designed to. Conditions that are as vastly different as arthritis and sleep apnea are all caused by our culturally influenced diet. It is understandable that a species that has spent 2 million years eating a certain way, and then is given a completely different menu within a couple thousand years will experience some problems with that menu.

There are a number of hunter/gatherer societies still around after all these generations, defying modern agricultural influences. The Inuit of North America, the Aborigines of Australia, and the Pygmies of Africa are all maintaining their numbers in defiance of much pressure from their surrounding countries. Most of the people in this type of society are remarkably fit and healthy. Despite the fact that they have no immunizations, no sanitation, and no modern medicine, they live healthy, full lives and generally have life expectancies longer than some industrialized nations.

Imagine if you take the naturally evolved diet of the hunter/gatherers and combined it with the medicine and sanitation of our modern world. You would have the healthiest lifestyle possible, and that is within all of our reach.

Some Initial Side Effects

To return to your natural way of eating, and thus the maximum health, there are a couple things you may experience. It's only fair to note that when you start the Evolution Diet, you may go through a 'hump' period of less energy and slight discomfort.

This is the natural process of weaning yourself off of the excess sugar and processed foods. Any dramatic switch in blood sugar from your normal routine may cause headaches. If you are accustomed to having copious amounts of glucose readily available for years prior to the diet, there stands to be a mild revolt from your body when you stop supplying it.

Additionally, any diet designed to take weight off will do a number of things initially. They will cause you to retain water and actually put a bit of water weight on you to start off. This may also be contributed by constipation. When you're lowering your calorie intake/expenditure rate, your body will want to hold on to any food you give it.

Don't fret though! Unlike using a drug or a get-thin-quick diet to lose weight, The Evolution Diet uses the natural progress of getting healthy. Any diet that drastically reduces your weight instantly is dangerous and will not last. The Evolution Diet could take a few weeks to start showing in your waistline, but other positive effects are instant and they are long-lasting! Once you have become acclimated to the diet you will begin to experience true health.

Some Positive Things To Look For

Though *all* the true benefits of eating what and how we were designed have not been documented, there are some obvious initial benefits that you can look for in your life right away!

High Energy: Most noticeably, you will experience a constant high level of energy throughout the day. You will not get the dramatic boosts in energy from a sugar or caffeine high and you will not get the dramatic lulls that tend to follow. You will experience the balanced energy of eating naturally.

Ideal Weight: Since you will be eating when your body tells you to and what nature tells you to, you will achieve your ideal weight. You will probably be eating more often, but you will be eating less densely concentrated foods. This should allow for a pleasurable dieting experience while you lose all those pounds!

Better Sleep: The main problem with people's physiology in today's society is due to their lack of quality sleep, and their lack of quality sleep is due to their unnatural diet. The Evolution Diet is specifically planned so that you don't give yourself mass quantities of energy before you want to go to sleep and it's designed to give you the added bonus of certain amino acids that aid in sleep. Also, you will be filling your stomach to capacity once a day (dinner);

this will tell your body that it's time to rest.

Relaxation: If you are stressed or irritated often, the Evolution Diet will help you relax. The constant, balanced energy level you will get throughout the day will lead to a more relaxed, less stressed person. In addition, the better sleep you will experience will also help you become more at ease other times of the day.

Better Physical Performance: When you begin to eat the way you were designed to eat, you will notice a marked improvement in your physical performance. This happens because you're producing energy when your body needs it and you're exercising when you are ready, not when it is convenient in your schedule.

More Enjoyment in Eating: If you're like most Evolution Dieters, you will experience a greater joy in eating. Since you are limited in your food selection at certain times of the day (meat throughout the day, for instance), you will learn to appreciate each food type more.

Better Dental Health: The process of constantly munching on things throughout the day, as specified in the Evolution Diet causes an increase in saliva output. This has been shown in many medical tests and is promoted by the use of sugarless chewing gum as a deterrent to cavities and gingivitis.

More Motivation to Exercise: Separating your diet into food groups designed for before and after exercise will help you motivate yourself to exercise. Of course, the energy boost of Energy Foods will help, but also, the reward system of a hearty High-Protein Meal after exercise will also give you motivation to work out.

Better Concentration: Throughout the day, you should expect to have better concentration and alertness due to the constant intake of moderate amounts of energy.

Better Immune System: When your body becomes accustomed to a consistent, natural way of eating, your immune system will benefit. All the energy that used to go to your stress-inducing diet can be concentrated on fighting off viruses and bacteria.

These benefits are great and they are immediate, but the true rewards are only seen in the long run. With the Evolution Diet, you will drastically reduce your chance of heart disease, obesity, diabetes, high blood pressure, stroke, depression, ADD, and food allergies.

These conditions are no joke and are directly caused by one's diet. Doctors all across the world are calling for better diets for the majority of people. If you choose to eat what and how you were designed, you can give yourself a better, and most likely a longer life.

A Better Life

You are on your way to becoming the person you've always wanted to be. You are going to use your body's naturally designed mechanics to work for you, not against you and you are going to live a better, healthier life for it.

The novelty of eating how our hunter/gatherer ancestors ate will wear off after a few weeks or months, but so will the pounds. And once you've gotten close to your ideal weight, you will not want to look back. The eating style will become second nature and you'll be able to fight off the urges for half a pizza at 10 P.M. or a giant-sized banana sundae right after a large dinner.

Unhealthy foods will begin to look unappetizing to you and you will relish your newfound will power. You will be able to turn down any food that's not appropriate because you'll know exactly what it does to your body and how you would feel as a result of it.

You'll know when to exercise and how to motivate yourself to exercise. When you are exercising, you won't feel sluggish and when you're done, you'll still have energy.

You now know that you have a greater chance of living longer, and those extra years that you live are going to be fun-filled. You won't dread going out into social events, or getting up out of bed any more. You will be excited to show your new self off and you'll have a deep sense of contentment inside, knowing that you've done one of the most difficult things in today's culture: you've gained optimal health.

The benefits are seemingly endless, and you're going to experience them all. You are on the way to becoming the ideal you, and all it took was a little reading! Congratulations, you have evolved!

Part Nine
Everything Else

"A beggar walked up to a woman who was just about to go into a coffee shop and exclaimed, "Lady, I haven't eaten in a week."

"Wow!" exclaimed the woman, "I wish I had your will power."
- Anonymous

| The Evolution Diet

breakfast and LoS Hi-Fi foods

Your body is designed to constantly eat these low sugar, high fiber foods (or LoS Hi-Fi foods) in small portions throughout the day. From when you get hungry in the morning until you eat dinner, you should be snacking on these foods.

LoS Hi-Fi foods are a source of consistent, balanced energy with some nutrition. A constant intake of small portions keeps your metabolism going at a high rate. Too much of these foods at one time, however will stifle your metabolism, overload your system with carbohydrates and cause fat gain.

Most grains and breads have minimal nutritious value, yet other LoS Hi-Fi foods, like vegetables and fruits are vital for our health. They provide the vitamins and minerals needed for life activities.

The best foods for daytime snacking are the ones with a low energy index (below 3) and a low protein index (below 2). These maximize the benefits of the LoS Hi-Fi foods. The higher the energy or protein index of a food, the worse it is for your constant snacking.

Energy breakdown for a typical LoS Hi-Fi food (Triscuit)

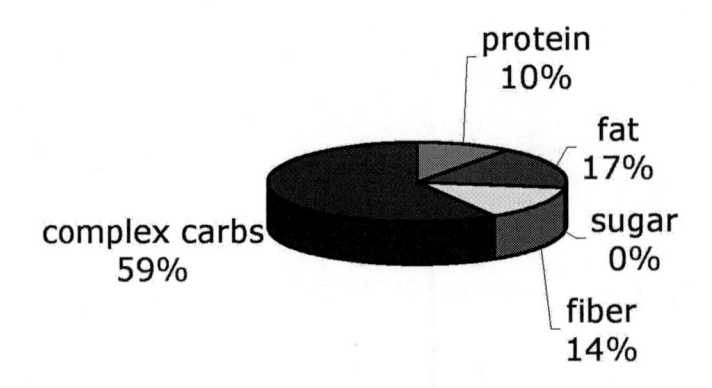

- protein 10%
- fat 17%
- sugar 0%
- fiber 14%
- complex carbs 59%

Source: CALORIE COUNTER

Note this is a limited list to give you a feel for the types of foods in this category. There are many other foods that belong to this category.

Everything Else | 103

LoS Hi-Fi foods (In order by Energy Index)

Grams	Food Name	Calories	Sugars	Total Carbs	Fiber	Protein	Energy Index	Protein Index
130	beans-black-canned	110	1	19	7	7	-0.354	2.541
247	soup-blackbean	116	0	19.8	4.4	5.6	0.156	1.102
10	lettuce-romaine	2	0	0.3	0.2	0.1	0.184	0.585
110	beans-green-snap	34	1.5	7.9	3.7	2	0.357	0.701
246	Hummus	435	1.1	49.5	9.8	12	0.386	1.234
245	milk-soy	120	1.2	11.4	3.2	9.2	0.519	2.044
62	cauliflower (cooked)	14	0.9	2.5	1.7	1.1	0.620	0.644
58	potato-baked	77	0	17.2	3.2	2.5	0.621	0.466
251	soup-clam chowder	176	0	21.8	1.5	10.9	0.665	1.659
120	celery-raw	17	2.2	3.6	1.9	0.8	0.755	-0.242
100	broccoli-raw	35	1.8	6.4	2.6	3	0.800	1.030
238	gravy-chicken	188	0.2	12.9	1	4.6	0.807	0.447
55	lettuce-iceberg	6	1	1.1	0.6	0.4	0.810	-0.204
631	pizza-whole-cheese,veggies, meat	1470	13	170.1	19	103.9	0.865	3.590
240	soup-beef with vegetables	170	1.6	19.6	1.4	11.7	0.942	1.741
696	spaghetti with meat sauce	640	17	92	12	23	1.069	0.354
255	salad-greek with feta	268	2	8.8	3.6	8.9	1.161	1.433
639	spaghetti with marinara	490	17	90	10	14	1.205	-0.295
240	soup-vegetable	122	4.4	19	1.2	3.5	1.218	-0.404
100	cereal-cheerios	393	3.3	73.3	10	10	1.250	-0.050
85	oatmeal-multigrain prepared	52	1.9	11.5	1.9	1.8	1.336	-0.436
160	egg noodles	213	0.5	39.7	1.8	7.6	1.375	-0.011
124	peas-green-sweet	70	4	11	3	4	1.565	0.145
30	salsa-tomato	10	1	2	0	0	1.667	-1.667
128	carrots	52	5.8	12.3	3.8	1.2	1.768	-1.289
133	sweet potato-raw	101	5.2	23.4	4	2.1	1.842	-1.270
100	bread-wheat	260	0	47	4.3	4	1.860	-1.159
200	chickpeas	728	0	45.2	8.8	10	2.091	-0.557
213	meatloaf-double sauced with gravy	360	3	19	1	23	2.235	3.472
231	burrito-bean	508	3	66	5	22.5	2.286	0.240
91	fish fillet-breaded-fried	211	0	15.4	0.5	13.3	2.308	3.121
245	milk-skim or fatfree	83	12.5	12.2	0	8.3	2.380	-0.118
100	bread-french	243	0	54.1	0	1.4	2.430	-2.212
248	sou-tomato	161	12.2	22.3	2.7	6.1	2.499	-1.204
100	bread-pita	275	0	56	2	9	2.590	-1.226
154	watermelon	46	9.5	11.6	0.6	0.9	2.757	-2.424
245	salad-fruit	74	16	19.3	2.5	0.9	2.812	-2.607
146	egg and cheese sandwich	340	2	25.9	1	15.6	2.849	1.003
158	fish sandwich-with tartar sauce	431	3	41	5	16.9	2.854	0.121
29	triscuit-ruduced fat	120	0	21	3	3	2.897	-1.641
151	Hummus and Feta Bagel	279	5	45	3	9	2.934	-1.436
200	rice-short-grain white	716	0	158.3	5.6	13	2.953	-2.224
402	Thai Chicken Pizza	663	16	89	5	40	2.993	0.103
28	triscuit-romsemary&olive	120	0	20	3	3	3.000	-1.684
100	pretzels-large soft	277	1.6	56.3	3.1	9.4	3.026	-1.608
240	milk-1% milkfat	130	15	16	0	11	3.042	-0.292
185	rice-long-grain brown	685	1.6	142.9	6.5	14.7	3.135	-2.224
130	chicken-boneless nuggets-fried	330	3	25	3	17.1	3.185	1.315
123	sandwich-Subway breakfast	320	3	34	3	15	3.285	-0.045
128	pistachio-dry roasted	731	10	35.4	13.2	27.3	3.391	2.273
146	pizza-slice-pepperoni	400	3	36.2	2.3	16.2	3.417	-0.228
177	cantaloupe	60	13.9	14.4	1.6	1.5	3.422	-2.955
100	pretzels-hard	381	0	79.2	2.8	9.1	3.496	-2.476
98	hotdog-plain	242	3	18	2	10.4	3.531	0.210
185	fish-battered fillet sandwich	520	4	44	2	18	3.589	-0.709
100	crackers-saltines	393	0	82	2.7	10.5	3.638	-2.497
97	tortilla-flour	330	1	45	2	8	3.649	-2.187
8	popcorn (air popped)	31	0.1	6.2	1.2	1	3.655	-2.226
185	orange	85	16.9	21.3	4.4	1.3	3.695	-3.368
9	rice cake-multigrain	35	0	7.2	0.3	0.8	3.849	-2.861
155	oatmeal-maple and brown sugar	157	12.6	31.1	2.8	3.7	4.062	-3.268
155	pineapple	74	14.4	19.6	2.2	0.8	4.069	-3.841
28.3	corn nuts	126	0.2	20.3	2	2.4	4.170	-3.132
125	apple	65	13	17.3	3	0.3	4.392	-4.291
258	peanutbutter-chunky	1520	20.1	54.4	17	64.7	4.527	3.540
232	cheese-cream	810	6.2	6.2	0	17.5	4.560	1.392
45	bread-white	132	2.1	24.5	1.1	4	4.692	-3.313
28	chips-tortilla	140	0	18	1	2	4.857	-3.896
106	hamburger with toppings	272	6.7	34.2	2.3	12.3	4.895	-2.149
11	popcorn (oil popped)	55	0.1	6.3	1.1	1	4.924	-3.572
248	apple juice	117	28.8	29	0.2	0.1	5.116	-5.098
225	banana	200	27.5	51.4	5.8	2.5	5.180	-4.841
248	lemonade	131	32.6	34.1	0.2	0.2	5.786	-5.752
250	smoothie café mocha	225	30.8	34	0	7.8	5.828	-4.506
28.3	Chex mix	120	1.6	18.4	1.6	3.1	6.140	-4.680
28	peanuts-salted	170	0.5	6	2	7	6.214	1.740

LoS Hi-Fi foods (In alphabetical order)

Grams	Food Name	Calories	Sugars	Total Carbs	Fiber	Protein	Energy Index	Protein Index
125	apple	65	13	17.3	3	0.3	4.392	-4.291
248	apple juice	117	28.8	29	0.2	0.1	5.116	-5.098
225	banana	200	27.5	51.4	5.8	2.5	5.180	-4.841
130	beans-black-canned	110	1	19	7	7	-0.354	2.541
110	beans-green-snap	34	1.5	7.9	3.7	2	0.357	0.701
100	bread-french	243	0	54.1	0	1.4	2.430	-2.212
100	bread-pita	275	0	56	2	9	2.590	-1.226
100	bread-wheat	260	0	47	4.3	4	1.860	-1.159
45	bread-white	132	2.1	24.5	1.1	4	4.692	-3.313
100	broccoli-raw	35	1.8	6.4	2.6	3	0.800	1.030
231	burrito-bean	508	3	66	5	22.5	2.286	0.240
177	cantaloupe	60	13.9	14.4	1.6	1.5	3.422	-2.955
128	carrots	52	5.8	12.3	3.8	1.2	1.768	-1.289
62	cauliflower (cooked)	14	0.9	2.5	1.7	1.1	0.620	0.644
120	celery-raw	17	2.2	3.6	1.9	0.8	0.755	-0.242
100	cereal-cheerios	393	3.3	73.3	10	10	1.250	-0.050
232	cheese-cream	810	6.2	6.2	0	17.5	4.560	1.392
28.3	Chex mix	120	1.6	18.4	1.6	3.1	6.140	-4.680
130	chicken-boneless nuggets-fried	330	3	25	3	17.1	3.185	1.315
200	chickpeas	728	0	45.2	8.8	10	2.091	-0.557
28	chips-tortilla	140	0	18	1	2	4.857	-3.896
28.3	corn nuts	126	0.2	20.3	2	2.4	4.170	-3.132
100	crackers-saltines	393	0	82	2.7	10.5	3.638	-2.497
146	egg and cheese sandwich	340	2	25.9	1	15.6	2.849	1.003
160	egg noodles	213	0.5	39.7	1.8	7.6	1.375	-0.011
91	fish fillet-breaded-fried	211	0	15.4	0.5	13.3	2.308	3.121
158	fish sandwich-with tartar sauce	431	3	41	5	16.9	2.854	0.121
185	fish-battered fillet sandwich	520	4	44	2	18	3.589	-0.709
238	gravy-chicken	188	0.2	12.9	1	4.6	0.807	0.447
106	hamburger with toppings	272	6.7	34.2	2.3	12.3	4.895	-2.149
98	hotdog-plain	242	3	18	2	10.4	3.531	0.210
246	Hummus	435	1.1	49.5	9.8	12	0.386	1.234
151	Hummus and Feta Bagel	279	5	45	3	9	2.934	-1.436
248	lemonade	131	32.6	34.1	0.2	0.2	5.786	-5.752
55	lettuce-iceberg	6	1	1.1	0.6	0.4	0.810	-0.204
10	lettuce-romaine	2	0	0.3	0.2	0.1	0.184	0.585
213	meatloaf-double sauced with gravy	360	3	19	1	23	2.235	3.472
240	milk-1% milkfat	130	15	16	0	11	3.042	-0.292
245	milk-skim or fatfree	83	12.5	12.2	0	8.3	2.380	-0.118
245	milk-soy	120	1.2	11.4	3.2	9.2	0.519	2.044
155	oatmeal-maple and brown sugar	157	12.6	31.1	2.8	3.7	4.062	-3.268
85	oatmeal-multigrain prepared	52	1.9	11.5	1.9	1.8	1.336	-0.436
185	orange	85	16.9	21.3	4.4	1.3	3.695	-3.368
258	peanutbutter-chunky	1520	20.1	54.4	17	64.7	4.527	3.540
28	peanuts-salted	170	0.5	6	2	7	6.214	1.740
124	peas-green-sweet	70	4	11	3	4	1.565	0.145
155	pineapple	74	14.4	19.6	2.2	0.8	4.069	-3.841
128	pistachio-dry roasted	731	10	35.4	13.2	27.3	3.391	2.273
146	pizza-slice-pepperoni	400	3	36.2	2.3	16.2	3.417	-0.228
631	pizza-whole-cheese,veggies, meat	1470	13	170.1	19	103.9	0.865	3.590
8	popcorn (air popped)	31	0.1	6.2	1.2	1	3.655	-2.226
11	popcorn (oil popped)	55	0.1	6.3	1.1	1	4.924	-3.572
58	potato-baked	77	0	17.2	3.2	2.5	0.621	0.466
100	pretzels-hard	381	0	79.2	2.8	9.1	3.496	-2.476
100	pretzels-large soft	277	1.6	56.3	3.1	9.4	3.026	-1.608
9	rice cake-multigrain	35	0	7.2	0.3	0.8	3.849	-2.861
185	rice-long-grain brown	685	1.6	142.9	6.5	14.7	3.135	-2.224
200	rice-short-grain white	716	0	158.3	5.6	13	2.953	-2.224
245	salad-fruit	74	16	19.3	2.5	0.9	2.812	-2.607
255	salad-greek with feta	268	2	8.8	3.6	8.9	1.161	1.433
30	salsa-tomato	10	1	2	0	0	1.667	-1.667
123	sandwich-Subway breakfast	320	3	34	3	15	3.285	-0.045
250	smoothie café mocha	225	30.8	34	0	7.8	5.828	-4.506
240	soup-beef with vegetables	170	1.6	19.6	1.4	11.7	0.942	1.741
247	soup-blackbean	116	0	19.8	4.4	5.6	0.156	1.102
251	soup-clam chowder	176	0	21.8	1.5	10.9	0.665	1.659
240	soup-vegetable	122	4.4	19	1.2	3.5	1.218	-0.404
248	sou-tomato	161	12.2	22.3	2.7	6.1	2.499	-1.204
639	spaghetti with marinara	490	17	90	10	14	1.205	-0.295
696	spaghetti with meat sauce	640	17	92	12	23	1.069	0.354
133	sweet potato-raw	101	5.2	23.4	4	2.1	1.842	-1.270
402	Thai Chicken Pizza	663	16	89	5	40	2.993	0.103
97	tortilla-flour	330	1	45	2	8	3.649	-2.187
28	triscuit-romsemary&olive	120	0	20	3	3	3.000	-1.684
29	triscuit-ruduced fat	120	0	21	3	3	2.897	-1.641
154	watermelon	46	9.5	11.6	0.6	0.9	2.757	-2.424

Notes:

High Protein Dinner Foods

These foods should be eaten after exercise, preferably in the evening a couple hours before sleep. Most high-protein foods (those with a Protein Index of 10 or higher) should be the main course and can be accompanied by moderately high protein foods (protein index between 2 and 10) and some low protein foods (protein index between 0 and 2). In order to calculate the percentage of your dinner that is protein you can use a simple guide: if all the foods are about the same amount of servings, add up all their protein indexes and add up all the energy indexes combined (if either number is negative, use .1). You should have a protein number and an energy number; add the two figures and divide the protein number by that number. That is your protein percentage.

Let's use a chicken burrito as an example. It's made up of basically three components: chicken, cheese, and the tortilla wrap.

chicken: Protein Index (PI): 27.029, Energy Index (EI): -3.877
cheese: PI: 20.190, EI: 2.667
wrap: PI -2.187, EI: 3.649

Protein = 27.029 + 20.190 - 2.187 = 45.032
Energy = (-3.877) + 2.667 + 2.187 = .977
Total = 46.009
Protein Percentage = 45.032 / 46.009 = 97.9% (That's really high!)

The Evolution Diet uses the Food Guide Pyramid as a guide for serving size. All of these are considered one serving:

1 slice bread
1 ounce of ready to eat cereal
1/2 cup of cooked cereal, rice, or pasta
1 cup of raw, leafy vegetables
1/2 cup other vegetables, cooked or chopped
1 medium apple, banana, orange
3/4 cup fruit juice
1 cup milk
2 oz cheese
2-3 oz of cooked lean meat, poultry, or fish
1/2 cup cooked dry beans or 1 egg counts as 1 oz of lean meat
2 tablespoons of peanutbutter or 1/3 cup of nuts count as 1 oz of lean meat.

Everything Else | 107

Some High Protein Foods also have a high energy index (e.g. beef jerky or peanutbutter) and should be eaten sparingly to avoid contradictory digestive reactions.

High protein foods are generally high in nutrition as well as protein. The fish that make up most of the top protein foods are high in essential fatty acids and essential amino acids. These foods are vital to our existence and should be eaten regularly.

The charts that follow are the high protein foods listed, first, in order of protein index and second, in alphabetical order.

Energy breakdown for a typical High Protein Food (Salmon)

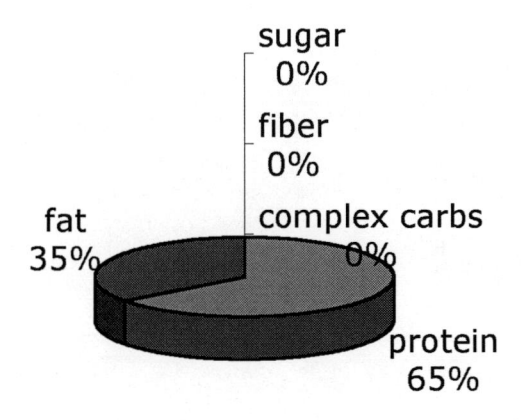

- sugar 0%
- fiber 0%
- complex carbs 0%
- protein 65%
- fat 35%

Source: CALORIE COUNTER

108 | The Evolution Diet

High Protein Foods (In order by Protein Index)

Grams	Food Name	Calories	Sugars	Total Carbs	Fiber	Protein	Energy Index	Protein Index
85	fish-tuna-bluefin	156	0	0	0	25.4	1.835	28.047
140	chicken-meat only-roasted	266	0	0	0	40.5	1.900	27.029
56	tuna-canned-in water	70	0	0	0	15	1.250	25.536
155	fish-salmon wild coho	285	0	0	0	42.4	1.839	25.516
85	pork loin	203	0	0	0	23.1	2.388	24.788
106	fish-swordfish-cooked	164	0	0	0	26.9	1.547	23.830
283	beef-select-cooked	824	0	0	0	74.1	2.912	23.272
154	fish-whitefish	265	0	0	0	37.7	1.721	22.760
101	fish-sea bass	125	0	0	0	23.9	1.238	22.426
180	fish-cod-atlantic-cooked	189	0	0	0	41.1	1.050	21.783
30	cheese-mozarella	80	0	0.5	0	8	2.667	20.190
178	fish-salmon-atlantic-cooked	367	0	0	0	39.3	2.062	20.017
85	shrimp	84	0	0	0	17.8	0.988	19.953
269	beef-ribs-broiled	920	0	0	0	59.8	3.420	18.810
136	sushi-swordfish	165	0	0	0	26.9	1.213	18.566
134	crab	130	0	0	0	25.9	0.970	18.358
198	sushi-salmon	362	0	0	0	39.4	1.828	18.071
85	fish-orange roughy	76	0	0	0	16	0.894	17.929
28.3	sushi-flounder	26	0	0	0	5.3	0.919	17.809
32	chicken wings- no sauce	103	0	0.8	0	8.4	3.219	17.781
136	fish-salmon-smoked	159	0	0	0	24.9	1.169	17.140
145	lobster	142	0	1.9	0	29.7	0.979	17.130
194	beans-black-raw	662	4.4	121	29.5	41.9	-13.624	16.608
240	cheese-brie	802	1.1	1.1	0	49.8	3.525	16.316
320	beef-corned	803	0	1.5	0	58.1	2.509	14.834
151	fish-sablefish	378	0	0	0	26	2.503	14.715
85	mussel-blue	146	0	6.3	0.2	20.2	1.716	11.933
84	chicken-fried breast with skin	218	0	7.6	0.3	20.9	2.591	10.472
243	eggs	357	1.9	1.9	0	30.6	1.782	9.897
126	tofu-raw	183	0	5.4	2.9	19.9	1.185	9.870
100	eggs-hard-boiled	155	0	1.1	0	12.5	1.550	9.711
243	egg-white-fresh	126	1.7	1.8	0	26.5	0.798	9.355
113	chicken-meat and skin-fried	313	0	10.7	0	26.6	2.770	9.321
226	cheese-cottage	203	0.7	8.2	0	31.1	1.022	9.075
226	cottage cheese	203	0.7	8.2	0	31.1	1.022	9.075
28.3	beef jerky	116	2.5	3.1	0.5	9.4	7.597	8.254
243	egg-yolk-fresh	782	1.4	8.7	0	38.5	3.449	8.218
15	eggs-omelet-just egg	23	0.1	0.1	0	1.6	1.800	8.200
87	fish-catfish-breaded-fried	199	0	7	0.6	15.7	2.271	7.729
73	chicken wings-with babrbeque sauce	160	3	5	0	14	3.836	7.546
61	eggs-egg beaters	30	1	1	0	6	1.148	7.303
256	beans-soy-raw	376	0	28.3	10.8	33.2	-0.354	6.513
205	tuna salad	383	1	19.3	2	32.9	1.985	6.281
150	cheese-feta	396	6.1	6.1	0	21.3	4.267	5.828
263	chili-beef and vegetable	339	2.9	42.9	19.2	13.4	-3.877	5.813
180	edemame (soybeans)	254	0	19.9	7.6	22.2	0.128	5.730
226	cottage cheese with fruit	219	5.4	10.4	0.5	24.2	1.920	5.413
259	hamburger-tripple patty with toppings	692	7	34.2	3	50	3.614	4.706
631	pizza-whole-cheese,veggies, meat	1470	13	170.1	19	103.9	0.865	3.590
258	peanutbutter-chunky	1520	20.1	54.4	17	64.7	4.527	3.540
213	meatloaf-double sauced with gravy	360	3	19	1	23	2.235	3.472
91	fish fillet-breaded-fried	211	0	15.4	0.5	13.3	2.308	3.121
130	beans-black-canned	110	1	19	7	7	-0.354	2.541
128	pistachio-dry roasted	731	10	35.4	13.2	27.3	3.391	2.273
245	milk-soy	120	1.2	11.4	3.2	9.2	0.519	2.044
240	soup-beef with vegetables	170	1.6	19.6	1.4	11.7	0.942	1.741
28	peanuts-salted	170	0.5	6	2	7	6.214	1.740
251	soup-clam chowder	176	0	21.8	1.5	10.9	0.665	1.659
255	salad-greek with feta	268	2	8.8	3.6	8.9	1.161	1.433
232	cheese-cream	810	6.2	6.2	0	17.5	4.560	1.392
130	chicken-boneless nuggets-fried	330	3	25	3	17.1	3.185	1.315
246	Hummus	435	1.1	49.5	9.8	12	0.386	1.234
247	soup-blackbean	116	0	19.8	4.4	5.6	0.156	1.102
100	broccoli-raw	35	1.8	6.4	2.6	3	0.800	1.030
146	egg and cheese sandwich	340	2	25.9	1	15.6	2.849	1.003
110	beans-green-snap	34	1.5	7.9	3.7	2	0.357	0.701
62	cauliflower (cooked)	14	0.9	2.5	1.7	1.1	0.620	0.644
10	lettuce-romaine	2	0	0.3	0.2	0.1	0.184	0.585
58	potato-baked	77	0	17.2	3.2	2.5	0.621	0.466
238	gravy-chicken	188	0.2	12.9	1	4.6	0.807	0.447
696	spaghetti with meat sauce	640	17	92	12	23	1.069	0.354
231	burrito-bean	508	3	66	5	22.5	2.286	0.240
98	hotdog-plain	242	3	18	2	10.4	3.531	0.210
124	peas-green-sweet	70	4	11	3	4	1.565	0.145
158	fish sandwich-with tartar sauce	431	3	41	5	16.9	2.854	0.121
402	Thai Chicken Pizza	663	16	89	5	40	2.993	0.103

High Protein Foods (In alphabetical order)

Grams	Food Name	Calories	Sugars	Total Carbs	Fiber	Protein	Energy Index	Protein Index
130	beans-black-canned	110	1	19	7	7	-0.354	2.541
194	beans-black-raw	662	4.4	121	29.5	41.9	-13.624	16.608
110	beans-green-snap	34	1.5	7.9	3.7	2	0.357	0.701
256	beans-soy-raw	376	0	28.3	10.8	33.2	-0.354	6.513
28.3	beef jerky	116	2.5	3.1	0.5	9.4	7.597	8.254
320	beef-corned	803	0	1.5	0	58.1	2.509	14.834
269	beef-ribs-broiled	920	0	0	0	59.8	3.420	18.810
283	beef-select-cooked	824	0	0	0	74.1	2.912	23.272
100	broccoli-raw	35	1.8	6.4	2.6	3	0.800	1.030
231	burrito-bean	508	3	66	5	22.5	2.286	0.240
62	cauliflower (cooked)	14	0.9	2.5	1.7	1.1	0.620	0.644
240	cheese-brie	802	1.1	1.1	0	49.8	3.525	16.316
226	cheese-cottage	203	0.7	8.2	0	31.1	1.022	9.075
232	cheese-cream	810	6.2	6.2	0	17.5	4.560	1.392
150	cheese-feta	396	6.1	6.1	0	21.3	4.267	5.828
30	cheese-mozarella	80	0	0.5	0	8	2.667	20.190
32	chicken wings- no sauce	103	0	0.8	0	8.4	3.219	17.781
73	chicken wings-with babrbeque sauce	160	3	5	0	14	3.836	7.546
130	chicken-boneless nuggets-fried	330	3	25	3	17.1	3.185	1.315
84	chicken-fried breast with skin	218	0	7.6	0.3	20.9	2.591	10.472
113	chicken-meat and skin-fried	313	0	10.7	0	26.6	2.770	9.321
140	chicken-meat only-roasted	266	0	0	0	40.5	1.900	27.029
263	chili-beef and vegetable	339	2.9	42.9	19.2	13.4	-3.877	5.813
226	cottage cheese	203	0.7	8.2	0	31.1	1.022	9.075
226	cottage cheese with fruit	219	5.4	10.4	0.5	24.2	1.920	5.413
134	crab	130	0	0	0	25.9	0.970	18.358
180	edemame (soybeans)	254	0	19.9	7.6	22.2	0.128	5.730
146	egg and cheese sandwich	340	2	25.9	1	15.6	2.849	1.003
243	eggs	357	1.9	1.9	0	30.6	1.782	9.897
61	eggs-egg beaters	30	1	1	0	6	1.148	7.303
100	eggs-hard-boiled	155	0	1.1	0	12.5	1.550	9.711
15	eggs-omelet-just egg	23	0.1	0.1	0	1.6	1.800	8.200
243	egg-white-fresh	126	1.7	1.8	0	26.5	0.798	9.355
243	egg-yolk-fresh	782	1.4	8.7	0	38.5	3.449	8.218
91	fish fillet-breaded-fried	211	0	15.4	0.5	13.3	2.308	3.121
158	fish sandwich-with tartar sauce	431	3	41	5	16.9	2.854	0.121
87	fish-catfish-breaded-fried	199	0	7	0.6	15.7	2.271	7.729
180	fish-cod-atlantic-cooked	189	0	0	0	41.1	1.050	21.783
85	fish-orange roughy	76	0	0	0	16	0.894	17.929
151	fish-sablefish	378	0	0	0	26	2.503	14.715
155	fish-salmon wild coho	285	0	0	0	42.4	1.839	25.516
178	fish-salmon-atlantic-cooked	367	0	0	0	39.3	2.062	20.017
136	fish-salmon-smoked	159	0	0	0	24.9	1.169	17.140
101	fish-sea bass	125	0	0	0	23.9	1.238	22.426
106	fish-swordfish-cooked	164	0	0	0	26.9	1.547	23.830
85	fish-tuna-bluefin	156	0	0	0	25.4	1.835	28.047
154	fish-whitefish	265	0	0	0	37.7	1.721	22.760
238	gravy-chicken	188	0.2	12.9	1	4.6	0.807	0.447
259	hamburger-tripple patty with toppings	692	7	34.2	3	50	3.614	4.706
98	hotdog-plain	242	3	18	2	10.4	3.531	0.210
246	Hummus	435	1.1	49.5	9.8	12	0.386	1.234
10	lettuce-romaine	2	0	0.3	0.2	0.1	0.184	0.585
145	lobster	142	0	1.9	0	29.7	0.979	17.130
213	meatloaf-double sauced with gravy	360	3	19	1	23	2.235	3.472
245	milk-soy	120	1.2	11.4	3.2	9.2	0.519	2.044
85	mussel-blue	146	0	6.3	0.2	20.2	1.716	11.933
258	peanutbutter-chunky	1520	20.1	54.4	17	64.7	4.527	3.540
28	peanuts-salted	170	0.5	6	2	7	6.214	1.740
124	peas-green-sweet	70	4	11	3	4	1.565	0.145
128	pistachio-dry roasted	731	10	35.4	13.2	27.3	3.391	2.273
631	pizza-whole-cheese,veggies, meat	1470	13	170.1	19	103.9	0.865	3.590
85	pork loin	203	0	0	0	23.1	2.388	24.788
58	potato-baked	77	0	17.2	3.2	2.5	0.621	0.466
255	salad-greek with feta	268	2	8.8	3.6	8.9	1.161	1.433
85	shrimp	84	0	0	0	17.8	0.988	19.953
240	soup-beef with vegetables	170	1.6	19.6	1.4	11.7	0.942	1.741
247	soup-blackbean	116	0	19.8	4.4	5.6	0.156	1.102
251	soup-clam chowder	176	0	21.8	1.5	10.9	0.665	1.659
696	spaghetti with meat sauce	640	17	92	12	23	1.069	0.354
28.3	sushi-flounder	26	0	0	0	5.3	0.919	17.809
198	sushi-salmon	362	0	0	0	39.4	1.828	18.071
136	sushi-swordfish	165	0	0	0	26.9	1.213	18.566
402	Thai Chicken Pizza	663	16	89	5	40	2.993	0.103
126	tofu-raw	183	0	5.4	2.9	19.9	1.185	9.870
205	tuna salad	383	1	19.3	2	32.9	1.985	6.281
56	tuna-canned-in water	70	0	0	0	15	1.250	25.536

Notes:

Notes:

High Energy Foods

When you are about to exercise (and you don't want to lose weight), you may want a little boost so that your muscles will perform at the top of their ability. High Energy Foods are full of instant energy because they are loaded with simple sugars.

It doesn't take long for your body to realize the affects of these foods, so you should eat them only when you need an immediate boost. This may happen when you're a little sluggish or tired. A small glass of orange juice may be just what the doctor ordered in the morning to accompany your LoS Hi-Fi breakfast, but a large bowl of extremely sugary cereal is not called for. When you take in too much of these foods, you will overload your system and most of it will go straight to fat.

Additionally, eating these foods at the wrong time can cause irritability, anxiousness, and soon after energy lulls and fatigue. Becoming dependent on these food also has its adverse effects. These are the foods that, when eaten often in mass quantities, result in diabetes and other diseases.

Eat these in extreme moderation before or during physical activity.

Energy breakdown for a typical High Energy Food (Grapes)

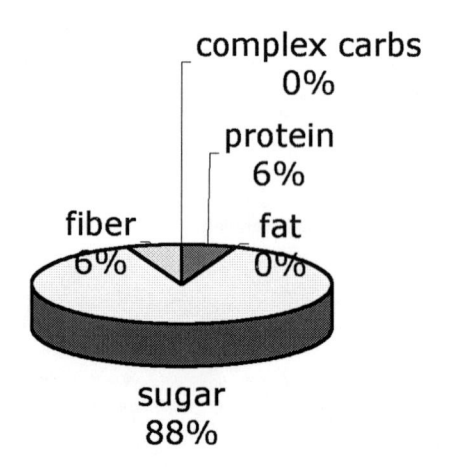

- complex carbs 0%
- protein 6%
- fiber 6%
- fat 0%
- sugar 88%

Source: CALORIE COUNTER

Everything Else | 113

High Energy Foods (In order by Energy Index)

Grams	Food Name	Calories	Sugars	Total Carbs	Fiber	Protein	Energy Index	Protein Index
27	cereal-peanutbutter crunch	120	10	22	1	2	19.111	-18.301
100	cereal-cinnamon toast crunch	440	34	79	4	5	17.360	-16.798
28.3	danish pastry	105	7.8	13.5	0.5	1.5	14.700	-13.781
60	granola	220	17	48	3	4.8	14.400	-13.511
28.3	cookies-oatmeal	127	7	19.4	0.8	1.8	14.291	-13.481
28.3	doughnut	119	6.4	14.1	0.4	1.4	13.228	-12.401
100	v-8 Splash	110	27	27	0	0	11.900	-11.900
146	trail mix	707	27	65.6	7	20.7	10.897	-8.316
30	cereal-multigrain cheerios	110	6	24	3	3	10.467	-9.356
100	cereal-raisin bran	317	33	79	13	8	9.610	-8.711
100	orange juice	105	20.9	24.5	0.5	1.5	9.400	-8.965
32	peanutbutter-creamy	190	3	7	2	8	9.188	-1.344
30	cereal-Wheaties	107	4.2	24.3	3	3	7.967	-6.868
30	wasabi peas	80	4	12	1	1	7.867	-7.200
30	crackers-tlc-original 7 grain	130	3	22	2	3	7.800	-6.600
70	macaroni and cheese-kraft	260	7	48	1	9	7.657	-6.021
28.3	beef jerky	116	2.5	3.1	0.5	9.4	7.597	8.254
28.3	potato chips	158	1.4	14.4	1	1.7	7.420	-6.434
129	cashews-oil roasted	749	6.5	38.9	4.3	21.7	7.248	-3.059
92	grapes	62	14.9	15.8	0.8	0.6	7.124	-6.884
65	corn bread	173	8	28.3	3	4.4	7.031	-5.766
694	Smoothie made with yogurt	480	102	110	4	10	6.478	-5.921
228	sweet potato-candied	203	35.1	47.7	5.7	2.2	6.478	-6.166
165	mango	107	24.4	28.1	3	0.8	6.345	-6.166

High Energy Foods (In alphabetical order)

Grams	Food Name	Calories	Sugars	Total Carbs	Fiber	Protein	Energy Index	Protein Index
28.3	beef jerky	116	2.5	3.1	0.5	9.4	7.597	8.254
129	cashews-oil roasted	749	6.5	38.9	4.3	21.7	7.248	-3.059
100	cereal-cinnamon toast crunch	440	34	79	4	5	17.360	-16.798
30	cereal-multigrain cheerios	110	6	24	3	3	10.467	-9.356
27	cereal-peanutbutter crunch	120	10	22	1	2	19.111	-18.301
100	cereal-raisin bran	317	33	79	13	8	9.610	-8.711
30	cereal-Wheaties	107	4.2	24.3	3	3	7.967	-6.868
28.3	cookies-oatmeal	127	7	19.4	0.8	1.8	14.291	-13.481
65	corn bread	173	8	28.3	3	4.4	7.031	-5.766
30	crackers-tlc-original 7 grain	130	3	22	2	3	7.800	-6.600
28.3	danish pastry	105	7.8	13.5	0.5	1.5	14.700	-13.781
28.3	doughnut	119	6.4	14.1	0.4	1.4	13.228	-12.401
60	granola	220	17	48	3	4.8	14.400	-13.511
92	grapes	62	14.9	15.8	0.8	0.6	7.124	-6.884
70	macaroni and cheese-kraft	260	7	48	1	9	7.657	-6.021
165	mango	107	24.4	28.1	3	0.8	6.345	-6.166
100	orange juice	105	20.9	24.5	0.5	1.5	9.400	-8.965
32	peanutbutter-creamy	190	3	7	2	8	9.188	-1.344
28.3	potato chips	158	1.4	14.4	1	1.7	7.420	-6.434
694	Smoothie made with yogurt	480	102	110	4	10	6.478	-5.921
228	sweet potato-candied	203	35.1	47.7	5.7	2.2	6.478	-6.166
146	trail mix	707	27	65.6	7	20.7	10.897	-8.316
100	v-8 Splash	110	27	27	0	0	11.900	-11.900
30	wasabi peas	80	4	12	1	1	7.867	-7.200

Notes:

Calorie Expenditures for Various Physical Activities for 1 Hour

BODY WEIGHT LB	97	110	123	137	159	163	176	190	203	216	229	242	255	269
Badminton	265	300	325	360	395	430	465	500	535	570	600	635	665	700
Baseball	210	225	240	255	270	285	290	305	320	335	350	365	380	395
Basketball	365	415	460	510	565	610	660	710	760	805	855	905	950	995
Competitive	390	445	500	550	600	655	710	760	810	865	910	960	1010	1065
Boxing	400	455	510	565	620	675	730	785	840	895	950	1005	1055	1110
Circuit Training	350	380	410	440	470	500	530	560	590	620	650	680	710	740
Cycle @ 12 mph	360	390	425	460	495	530	565	600	635	670	705	740	775	810
Racing	450	510	570	630	690	750	810	870	930	990	1050	1110	1170	1230
Dancing	270	295	320	345	370	395	420	445	470	495	520	545	570	595
Golf	230	260	290	320	350	380	410	440	470	500	530	560	590	620
Horse Riding	240	275	310	345	370	405	440	475	510	545	580	615	650	685

BODY WEIGHT LB	97	110	123	137	159	163	176	190	203	216	229	242	255	269
Rowing Crew	600	660	720	780	830	890	940	1000	1060	1120	1180	1235	1295	1345
Running @ 6.5 mph	425	480	535	590	650	705	760	820	875	930	985	1045	1100	1160
@ 10 mph	620	690	765	835	900	965	1035	1100	1170	1235	1300	1365	1430	1495
Skating (inline)	250	285	320	355	380	410	445	480	515	550	590	625	660	700
Skiing (piste)	295	335	375	415	455	495	535	575	615	655	695	735	775	815
Soccer	355	400	445	490	535	580	625	670	715	760	805	850	895	940
Squash	515	580	645	710	785	850	915	980	1045	1110	1175	1240	1305	1370
Swimming Slow	230	260	290	320	350	380	410	440	470	500	530	560	590	620
Fast laps	400	445	490	535	580	625	670	705	750	795	840	885	930	975
Tennis social	300	340	375	415	455	490	530	570	605	645	680	720	760	795
Weight Training	350	395	440	485	530	575	620	665	710	755	800	845	890	935
Walking 5 kph.	200	220	240	260	280	300	320	340	360	380	400	420	440	460

Note: Figures are just estimates and may not be completely accurate. Muscle mass and activity level play a part in determining the actual calorie expenditure.

Recipes

Due to the inconsistent nature of the sources of these recipes, some exact nutritional information is not available. Each item does, however fit into the category under which it is listed based on its ingredients.

Low Sugar, High Fiber Foods
(LoS Hi-Fi foods to be eaten throughout the day in small quantities)

Blueberry Oat Bran Muffins
Energy Index: 5.311   Protein Index: 4.218
Serves: 12 (1 muffin) servings.
Working Time: 10 minutes.
Total Time: 30 minutes.

2 tsp. baking powder
2 tbsp. canola oil
1/4 cup fat free egg substitute
1/4 cup honey
1/2 cup oat bran
1 cup reduced fat buttermilk
1 cup rolled oats
1 cup unbleached all purpose flour
1 1 2/ cups unsweetened frozen blueberries, thawed

1 Preheat the oven to 375°F.
2 Spray 12 muffin tin cups with nonstick cooking spray or line them with paper liners.
3 In a small bowl stir together the buttermilk, honey, oil, and egg substitute.
4 In a large bowl stir together the oats, oat bran, flour, and baking powder, and make a well in the center. Pour in the milk mixture and the blueberries and stir just until combined; do not overmix.
5 Divide the batter among the muffin cups and bake 20 to 25 minutes, or until a toothpick inserted into the center of a muffin comes out clean and dry.

Calories: 141
Protein: 4g
Carbohydrate: 24g
Dietary Fiber: 2g
Total Fat: 4g
Saturated Fat: 1g
Cholesterol: 1mg
Sodium: 99mg.

Garbanzo Pita Pockets
Energy Index: 2.998   Protein Index: -0.743
Yields: 4 (1 pita) servings.
Working Time: 10 minutes.
Total Time: 15 minutes.

1 (15 oz.) can reduced sodium garbanzo beans, drained and rinsed
1 (6 oz.) jar marinated artichoke hearts, quartered, liquid reserved
1 tbsp. black olives, sliced
1 clove garlic, minced
1 small green bell pepper, diced
1 tbsp. green olives, sliced
2 cups lettuce, shredded
1 tsp. Nutrific Cuisine Garden Herb Salt Free Spice Blend
1 small red bell pepper, diced
1 small red onion, thinly sliced
2 tbsp. red wine vinegar
4 large slices pita bread

Calories: 367, Protein: 15g, Carbohydrate: 67g, Dietary Fiber: 15g, Total Fat: 8g, Saturated Fat: 0g, Cholesterol: 0mg, Sodium: 582mg.

Note - For each teaspoon of the Garden Herb Spice Blend, you may substitute: 1/4 tsp. basil, 1/4 tsp. marjoram, 1/4 tsp. dill weed, and 1/4 tsp. black pepper.

1 In a large bowl, combine the garbanzo beans, peppers, onion, garlic, olives, artichokes, and their liquid, vinegar, and seasoning.
2 Mix well; set aside.
3 Slice off the top third of each pita bread; open the bread to

form a pocket.
4 Place an equal amount of lettuce in each pita and fill with the garbanzo filling.

Couscous with Tomatoes, Basil and Lentils
Energy Index: 4.870   Protein Index: .012

1 Tbsp (15mL) olive oil
3 cloves garlic, minced
1 1/2 cups (360mL) vegetable juice cocktail, (V8 or seasoned tomato juice)
1 1/2 cups (360mL) water
1 cup (230g) lentils, uncooked, rinsed and drained
1 bay leaf, broken in half
1/2 tsp (3g) salt (sea salt if on a corn-free diet*)
1/2 tsp (2g) freshly ground pepper
1 cup (200g) couscous, uncooked
1 tomato, chopped
1/2 cup (20g) fresh basil leaves, chopped

1. In a medium-sized pot, heat oil until hot and sauté garlic until tender.
2. Stir in vegetable juice, water, lentils, bay leaf, salt and pepper.
3. Bring to a boil and reduce heat to low.
4. Cover and simmer for 30 to 40 minutes, or until lentils are soft but not mushy.
5. Remove pot from heat and discard bay leaf. Stir in couscous, tomato and basil.
6. Cover and let stand for 5 minutes or until the couscous is soft.
7. Uncover and fluff with a fork to separate the grains.

* Allergy notes: People following a corn-free diet should avoid iodized salt since it contains dextrose, which should be avoided by those allergic to corn.

Nutrition Facts
Calories: 383
Total Fat: 4g
% Calories from fat: 9%
Protein: 20g

Carbohydrate: 67g
Cholesterol: 0mg
Sodium: 527mg

Inca Platter
Energy Index: 2.341   Protein Index: 3.444

Quinoa salad:

1 cup (200g) quinoa, well rinsed
1 cup (150g) frozen corn kernels, thawed
Juice of one lemon
1 Tbsp (15mL) olive oil
2 to 3 scallions, minced
Salt and black pepper, to taste

Bean salad:

1 16-ounce (455g) can pinto beans, drained
1 cup (200g) diced tomato
1 Tbsp (15mL) apple cider
1/4 cup (10g) chopped parsley or cilantro
Freshly ground black pepper, to taste

Garnishes:

Pumpkin seeds
Black olives
1 red bell pepper, cut into strips

1. Boil 2 cups water (480mL) in a saucepan.
2. Add the quinoa and simmer, covered, for 15 minutes.
3. When done, fluff with a fork and transfer to a bowl.
4. Combine quinoa with remaining ingredients for the quinoa salad.
5. While the quinoa cooks, toss the bean salad ingredients in another bowl.
6. To assemble, spread quinoa salad evenly on a platter. Leave a well in the center and mound bean salad into the well.
7. Sprinkle with pumpkin seeds.
8. Arrange olives and pepper strips around the edge.

Nutrition Facts
Calories: 283
Fat: 6g
% fat calories: 19%
Cholesterol: 0mg
Fiber: 14g

Falafel
Energy Index: 4.781   Protein Index: 1.104

1 can (15 ounces or 425g) garbanzo beans, rinsed and drained
1 medium onion, coarsely chopped
1/4 cup (10g) packed parsley leaves
2 cloves garlic, minced
1/2 tsp (1g) ground cumin
3/4 tsp (1.5g) dried oregano leaves
2—3 tsp (10–15mL) lemon juice
Salt and pepper, to taste
1 cup (115g) dry plain bread crumbs, divided
1/4 cup (40g) chopped raisins
1 egg yolk
Olive oil cooking spray

Tomato-Cucumber Relish:

1/2 cup (100g) chopped tomato
1/2 cup (75g) chopped cucumber
1/3 cup (80g) fat-free plain yogurt
1/2 tsp (1g) dried mint leaves (optional)
Salt and pepper, to taste

1. Process garbanzo beans, onion, parsley, garlic, cumin and oregano in a food processor until smooth; season to taste with lemon juice, salt, and pepper.
2. Stir in 1/2 cup (60g) bread crumbs, raisins and egg yolk.
3. Form bean mixture into 16 patties, using about 1 1/2 Tbsp (25mL) for each.
4. Coat patties with remaining 1/2 cup (60g) bread crumbs.
5. Spray large skillet with cooking spray; heat over medium heat

until hot.
6. Cook falafel over medium heat until browned on the bottom, 2 to 3 minutes.
7. Spray tops of falafel with cooking spray and turn; cook until browned on the bottom, 2 to 3 minutes.
8. Arrange 4 falafel on each plate; serve with Tomato-Cucumber Relish.

To make Tomato-Cucumber Relish:

Combine tomato, cucumber, yogurt and mint leaves in small bowl.
Season to taste with salt and pepper.

* Allergy notes: People following a corn-free diet should avoid iodized salt since it contains dextrose, which should be avoided by those allergic to corn.

Nutrition Facts
Calories: 311
Fat: 4g
% fat calories: 12%
Cholesterol: 54mg
Carbohydrate: 58g
Protein: 12g
Fiber: 7g
Sodium: 575mg

Bowl 'a' Granola
Energy Index: 8.311   Protein Index: -2.237

41/2 cups (385g) rolled oats
1/4 cup (30g) wheat bran
1/2 cup (60g) wheat germ
1/4 cup (30g) nuts or seeds (try a combo such as sunflower or sesame seeds and walnuts)
1/2 cup (120mL) honey
1/4 cup apple juice
1/2 cup (75g) assorted, chopped dried fruit such as apricots,

apples or figs
2 Tbsp (30mL) canola oil
2 tsp (4g) cinnamon

1. Preheat oven to 350°F (175°C). Coat a 9x13-inch (23x33cm) pan with nonstick cooking spray.
2. In a large bowl, mix together oats, bran, germ, nuts and cinnamon.
3. Blend honey, canola oil and juice. Add mixture to oats and stir until well-coated.
4. Spread granola onto a baking sheet and cook 25 minutes, stirring a few times so that granola browns evenly.
5. Remove from oven and let the granola cool on the baking sheet for 10 minutes.
6. Add dried fruit when mixture cools. Store in an air-tight container.

Nutrition Facts
Calories: 488
Fat: 12g
% fat calories: 22%
Cholesterol: 0mg
Carbohydrate: 85g
Fiber: 10g

Fresh Pineapple Fruit Salad
Energy Index: 6.381   Protein Index: -2.252
Working Time: 10 min, plus chilling time.

1 whole pineapple
1 papaya, peeled, seeded, cut into chunks
1/4 lb. seedless grapes
1 apple, peeled cored and cut into chunks
1/4 cup pecan halves
1 banana, sliced
1/4 cup lime juice
1 lime, quartered, as garnish

1. Cut pineapple lengthwise into quarters.

2 Cut away and discard core.
3 Remove pineapple flesh by carefully cutting between it and outer skin of pineapple to use the shell for a salad bowl.
4 Cut pineapple into chunks and combine with remaining ingredients, except lime wedges, in a bowl.
5 Gently toss and **chill** if desired.
6 Serve fruit salad in a pineapple shell topped with lime garnish.

Black Beans in Pita Pockets
Energy Index: 3.311   Protein Index: 1.297
Working Time: 10 min, Marinate: 30 min.

1-1/2 lbs. canned black beans, rinsed and drained
2 Tbs. chopped pimento
2 Tbs. parsley
1 Tbs. plus 1 tsp. olive oil
2 Tbs. lemon juice
1-1/2 Tbs. water
1/4 tsp. dry mustard
1 clove garlic, minced
4 pita pocket breads, warm and cut in half

Combine beans, pimento and parsley in a salad bowl.
Combine remaining ingredients, except pitas, in a jar with a tight-fitting lid.
Add salt and pepper to taste.
Shake vigorously.
Pour dressing over beans.
Set aside 30 minutes.
Divide equally and stuff into pita breads.

Baja Black Beans, Corn and Rice
Energy Index: 3.912   Protein Index: 2.549

6 cups (1.2kg) brown rice, cooked
1 2/3 cups (425g) black beans, (one 15-ounce can), rinsed and drained
1 2/3 cups (425g) corn, (one 15-ounce can), drained
4 fresh tomatoes, diced
1/2 cup (90g) red onion, chopped
1/2 cup (20g) cilantro, chopped

1 jalapeno chile pepper, seeded and diced
2 Tbsp (30mL) fresh lime juice
1 Tbsp (15mL) olive oil
1/2 tsp (3g) salt
1/4 tsp (1g) freshly ground black pepper
2 dashs hot sauce

1. Cook brown rice.
2. In a medium bowl, combine black beans, corn, tomatoes, onion, cilantro, jalapeno, lime juice, oil, salt, pepper, and hot sauce.
3. To serve, place a scoop of hot rice in a bowl or on a plate, top with a generous scoop of the black bean mixture. Stir together before eating.

Nutrition Facts
Calories: 499
Total Fat: 6g
% Calories from fat: 10%
Protein: 19g
Carbohydrate: 96g
Cholesterol: 0mg
Sodium: 2193mg

Garbanzo and Zucchini Soup
Energy Index: 0.591   Protein Index: 2.372

2 Tbsp (30mL) olive oil
1 medium onion, chopped
1 clove garlic, chopped
3 Tbsp (7g) parsley, chopped
3 Tbsp (7g) fresh basil, chopped
2 medium zucchini, whole
1 can (425g) garbanzo beans, (15 ounces)
1 tsp (6g) salt (sea salt if on a corn-free diet*)
3 cups (720mL) water
1 bunch beet greens or other mild flavored greens
Pepper to taste
4 tsp (10g) Parmesan cheese*, grated, optional

1. In a large soup pot, heat olive oil and add onion.
2. Sauté onion until transparent.
3. Add garlic, parsley and basil and cook for a few minutes more.
4. Add zucchini and cook just until the squash is tender, stirring occasionally. Add garbanzo beans, salt, and water and bring to a boil.
5. Turn heat down and cook over medium heat for about 20 minutes.
6. Meanwhile, place greens in a sink full of water and swish around to thoroughly wash them.
7. Drain water, and shake the greens to partially dry them.
8. Place them on a cutting board and cut the leaves into pieces measuring approximately 2x1/2 inches (5x1.5cm).
9. Cook for about 10 more minutes, until the greens have cooked down.
10. Add fresh ground pepper, and serve with about 1 tsp (3g) of Parmesan cheese per serving.
11. Add the greens to the soup pot and stir well.

* Allergy notes: People following a corn-free diet should avoid iodized salt since it contains dextrose, which should be avoided by those allergic to corn. The egg protein lysozyme is an unlabeled additive in some cheeses. People allergic to eggs should eliminate any cheese in this recipe.

Nutrition Facts
Calories: 279
Total Fat: 11g
% Calories from fat: 32%
Protein: 12g
Carbohydrate: 37g
Cholesterol: 1mg
Sodium: 589mg

Healthy Cajun Beans and Rice
Energy Index: 5.142   Protein Index: 3.722
Working Time: 10 min, Cook: 15 min.

Recipes | 129

1 Tbs. vegetable oil
1/2 lb. turkey sausage, sliced into 1/2 inch thick slices
1 medium onion, chopped
1 medium green bell pepper, chopped
2 cloves garlic, minced
6 cups cooked rice
1 lb. canned kidney beans, drained and rinsed
1 lb. canned navy beans, drained and rinsed
3-1/2 cups canned stewed tomatoes, Cajun-style
1 tsp. oregano
1/2 tsp. hot pepper sauce
1 cup green onions, thinly sliced

1. Heat oil in large skillet over medium-high heat until hot.
2. Add sausage, onion, green pepper, and garlic.
3. Cook, stirring 7-10 minutes, or until sausage is browned and onion is tender.
4. Add rice, kidney beans, navy beans, tomatoes, oregano, and hot pepper sauce.
5. Cook and stir 2-3 minutes more until well blended and thoroughly heated.
6. Sprinkle with green onions and serve immediately.

Courtesy American Dry Bean Board.

Per serving: calories 775
fat 10.7g, 12% calories from fat
cholesterol 35mg
protein 32.8g
carbohydrates 138.1g
 fiber 14.4g
sugar 17.3g
sodium 942mg

Squash and Yam Soup
Energy Index: 6.388   Protein Index: -4.271
Working Time: 15 min, Cook: 20 min.

2 lbs. butternut squash, peeled, seeded and cut into 1 inch pieces
3/4 lb. yams, peeled and cut into 1 inch pieces
1 Tbs. unsalted butter

1 onion, chopped
2 cloves garlic, minced
1 Tbs. fresh ginger, peeled and minced
1/2 tsp. cinnamon
1/4 tsp. ground ginger
1/8 tsp. red pepper flakes
4 cups vegetable stock
2 Tbs. pure maple syrup
2 Tbs. orange marmalade

1. Place squash and yams in a steamer basket over boiling water.
2. Cover saucepan and **steam** 20 minutes or until tender.
3. Remove steamer basket and set aside.
4. Melt butter in a heavy nonstick skillet over medium high heat.
5. Sauté onions 7-8 minutes or until golden brown.
6. Stir in garlic and fresh ginger and sauté 1 minute.
7. Stir in cinnamon, ground ginger and chili pepper flakes.
8. Add half the stock to skillet, stirring with a wooden spoon to deglaze.
9. Working in batches, purée onion mixture, squash, yams and maple syrup in a blender or food processor until smooth.
10. Transfer purée to a saucepan.
11. Add remaining stock, salt and pepper to taste.
12. Cook until heated throughout.
13. Serve with a dollop of orange marmalade.

Per serving: calories 310
fat 4.0g, 11% calories from fat
cholesterol 8mg
protein 4.6g
carbohydrates 69.6g
fiber 12.0g
sugar 22.2g
sodium 499mg

Strawberry Banana Bar
Energy Index: 7.001   Protein Index: -2.160
 Serves: 96   (4 long pans)

16   Eggs

4 C	Unsweetened Applesauce
2 C	Oil
6 C	Brown Sugar
2T +2 tsp	Vanilla Extract
12C	Frozen Bananas, MASHED
8 C	Frozen Strawberries MASHED
16 C	Whole Wheat Flour
2 T + 2 tsp	Baking Soda
1/2 C	Ground Cinnamon

1. Preheat oven to 375 degrees.
2. In large bowl, mix eggs, applesauce, oil, brown sugar, vanilla and bananas.
3. Combine dry ingredients and stir into banana mixture.
4. Stir in mashed strawberries.
5. Bane for 20 min. or until top springs back when pressed lightly.

Wheat Germ Sesame Bread
Energy Index: 0.946   Protein Index: 1.884
 1 loaf Change size or US/metric
Working Time : 1 hour 30 minutes 1 hr prep

1 cup **water**
3 tablespoons **vegetable oil**
3 tablespoons **honey**
1 **egg**
1 teaspoon **salt**
3 tablespoons **wheat germ**
1 1/2 tablespoons **sesame seeds**
1 cup **whole-wheat flour**
2 cups **bread flour**
1 1/2 teaspoons **dry yeast**

Add ingredients following manufacturer's recommendations.
can be baked in the machine.
or use dough setting.
remove and form into loaf.
place in oiled bread pan.
rise until doubled.
bake in 375 degree oven for 30 minutes.

Hummus
3 cups Change size or US/metric
Working Time: 10 minutes 10 mins prep

2 (15 ounces) cans **garbanzo beans** (reserve juice)
5 cloves **garlic**
6 ounces **fresh lemon juice**
1/2 cup **tahini**
1 1/2 teaspoons **salt**
1 teaspoon smoked **paprika**
 extra virgin olive oil

1. Food processor: process garlic, add remaining ingredients and pulse to desired consistency (thin with juice from can if needed).
2. Put hummus in a bowl, sprinkle with a drizzle of olive oil and smoked paprika.

Crunchy New Potatoes
Energy Index: 2.450   Protein Index: -0.087
4-5 servings Change size or US/metric
Working Time: 55 minutes 20 mins prep

16 small new **red potatoes**
1 (1 ounce) package dry **hidden valley ranch dressing mix**
2 cups coarsely crushed **corn flakes**
1/2 cup melted **butter**

1. Preheat oven to 400 degrees.
2. Cook potatoes in boiling water until tender—about 10 minutes.
3. Drain and let cool slightly.
4. Peel.
5. Mix salad dressing mix and corn flakes in plate.
6. Dip potatoes in melted butter and then roll in cornflake mixture.
7. Place in greased baking dish, in single layer, and bake 20-25 minutes or until golden brown.

La Batisserrie French Bread
Energy Index: 2.345   Protein Index: -1.869
 1 loaf Change size or US/metric
Working Time: 10 minutes 10 mins prep This makes a 1 1/2 lb. loaf.

4 cups **bread flour**
1 1/3 cups **water**
1 teaspoon **salt**
1 teaspoon **sugar**
2 1/2 teaspoons **active dry yeast**

Use the french bread or basic bread setting on your machine. Wrap in a paper bag to store.

Banana Pecan Whole Wheat Mini Muffins
Energy Index: 5.334   Protein Index: -2.443
 3 dozen mini muffins Change size or US/metric
Working Time: 30 minutes 15 mins prep

1/2 cup **butter**
1/2 cup **sugar**
1 cup **oat bran**
1 **egg**
2 tablespoons **water**
1 1/2 cups mashed **bananas**
1 1/2 cups **whole wheat pastry flour**
2 teaspoons **baking powder**
1/2 teaspoon **salt**
1/2 teaspoon **baking soda**
1 teaspoon **vanilla**
1/2 cup chopped **pecans**

1 Preheat the oven to 350 degrees.
2 Spray your mini muffin pans with non stick spray.
3 Beat the butter and sugar together.
4 Add the egg and mix well.

5 Then add the oat bran and mix well.
6 In a separate container combine the mashed banana with the 2 tablespoons water.
7 Mix the fry ingredients together.
8 Add the banana mix to the butter alternatively with the mixed dry ingredients.
9 Mix well.
10 Add the vanilla and the pecans.
11 Bake for about 15 minutes or until the muffins start to brown.

Soft Pumpernickel Bread (abm).
Energy Index: 3.811   Protein Index: -1.934
1 loaf   Change size or US/metric
Working Time: 10 minutes   10 mins prep

1 cup lukewarm **water**
3 tablespoons **honey**
1 1/2 tablespoons **molasses**
1 tablespoon **butter**
2 teaspoons **salt**
3/4 cup **rye flour**
1 1/2 cups **bread flour**
3/4 cup **whole-wheat flour**
2 teaspoons **active dry yeast**

1 Add ingredients to bread machine in order as per your manufacturer's directions.
2 Select dough setting.
3 Place in greased loaf pan, cover and let rise for 30 minutes.
4 Bake at 375° for 25 to 30 minutes.
5 Remove from pan and let cool on wire rack.

Roasted Salted Sunflower Seed
Energy Index: 2.091   Protein Index: 0.214
Working Time: 1 hour 30 minutes   1 hr prep

1 cup **sunflower seeds**
2 quarts **water**

1/2 cup **salt**
1 cup Change size or US/metric

1. Place water and salt in a saucepan.
2. Rinse sunflower seeds and remove any plant or flower head matter.
3. Add sunflower seeds to water& salt in pan.
4. Bring water to a boil, then turn down to simmer.
5. Simmer 1 to 1 1/2 hours.
6. When done, strain water& seeds through colander& allow seeds to dry
7. on paper toweling. Do not rinse.
8. Preheat oven to 325 degrees.
9. Spread seeds on a cookie sheet& bake for 25 to 30 minutes.
10. Stir frequently.
11. Remove from oven when seeds are slightly browned& fragrant.

NOTE: for salt free seeds, simply eliminate the first 7 steps& go straight into oven preparation (Step 8).

Cinnamon Applesauce Yeast Bread
Energy Index: 4.197   Protein Index: 1.455
Working Time: 10 minutes 10 mins prep

1 1/4 cups **applesauce**
2 tablespoons **butter**
1 1/2 tablespoons **sugar**
1 teaspoon **salt**
1 teaspoon **cinnamon**
1 cup **whole-wheat flour**
2 cups **bread flour**
1 1/2 teaspoons **active dry yeast**
1 loaf Change size or US/metric

1. Add all ingredients to bread machine in order given by the manufacturer.
2. Check the dough after 5 minutes of kneading; if too wet, add more flour.

Savory Zucchini Cheese Bread
Energy Index: 1.884 Protein Index: 3.804
Working Time: 1 hour 20 mins prep

1 cup chopped **onions**
1/4 cup **butter**
2 1/2 cups **Bisquick**
1/2 teaspoon **dried parsley**
1/2 teaspoon **dried basil**
1/2 teaspoon **dried thyme**
1/4 cup **milk**
3 **eggs**
1 1/2 cups shredded **zucchini**
1 cup shredded **cheddar cheese**
3/4 cup toasted chopped **almonds**
1 round loaf Change size or US/metric

1 In saucepan, melt butter.
2 Cook onion until soft.
3 Cool slightly.
4 Mix onion mixture, bisquick, herbs, milk and eggs; beat on high for one minute.
5 Stir in remaining ingredients.
6 Spread in greased and floured 9" round pan.
7 Bake at 400 degrees for about 40 minutes until wooden pick comes out clean.
8 Cool slightly and remove from pan.

Old-timey Whole Wheat Bread
Energy Index: 1.864 Protein Index: -1.147
Working Time: 2 hours 40 minutes 2 hrs prep

5 cups **flour**
2 packages **dry yeast**
2 3/4 cups **water**
1/2 cup **brown sugar**
1/4 cup **shortening**
1 tablespoon **salt**

3 cups **whole-wheat flour**
2 loaves Change size or US/metric

1. Mix 3 1/2 cup flour and yeast.
2. Heat water, brown sugar, shortening, and salt until warm (115-120 degrees) stirring to melt shortening.
3. Add to dry mix in bowl.
4. Beat 1/2 minute on low; 3 minutes on high.
5. Stir in whole wheat flour and enough other flour to make moderately stiff dough.
6. Knead until smooth and elastic (10-12 min.) Place in large greased bowl, turn.
7. Cover, let rise until double (1 hr).
8. Punch down, divide in 1/2, cover; let rest 10 minutes.
9. Shape into loaves and place in 2 greased 9x5 loaf pans.
10. Cover, let rise until double (45 min.) Bake at 375 degrees for 40-45 minutes.

Tennessee Corn Bread
Energy Index: 2.054   Protein Index: -2.895
Working Time: 1 hour 20 minutes 20 mins prep

2 tablespoons **butter** or solid veggie **shortening**
2 cups **white cornmeal**
1/2 cup **all-purpose flour** (sifted before measuring)
1/2 cup **sugar**
1/2 teaspoon **salt**
1 teaspoon **baking powder**
1/2 teaspoon **baking soda**
2 cups **buttermilk**
1 **egg**, beaten
1 loaf Change size or US/metric

1. Prepare Corn Bread: Heat oven to 350°.
2. Put butter in 9x5x2 inch loaf pan.
3. Place in oven to let butter melt.
4. Meanwhile, sift together in large bowl cornmeal, flour, sugar, salt, baking powder and baking soda.

5. Add buttermilk and egg to cornmeal-flour mixture.
6. Remove loaf pan from oven and pour hot melted butter into cornmeal mixture.
7. Set loaf pan aside to cool.
8. Using a wooden spoon, mix corn bread batter only until all dry ingredients are moistened.
9. Thoroughly grease the inside of the cooled loaf pan with solid vegetable shortening.
10. This corn bread can stick to the pan so be SURE YOU GREASE THE PAN VERY HEAVILY.
11. If possible, use a pan with a nonstick finish.
12. Pour bread batter into prepared pan and put it on the center rack of the preheated oven.
13. Bake for 1 hour or until a cake tester comes out clean.
14. Bread should be very light golden brown.
15. Remove pan from oven and immediately turn bread out onto a breadboard.
16. Let cool about 5 min.
and cut into thick slices.
17. Serve with plenty of butter or honey butter (makes 1 loaf of bread).

High Protein Dinner Foods
(Foods that should be eaten in large quantities 1-2 hours after exercise and 3-4 hours before sleep)

The Holy Crêpe!® Peace, Love, and Ham ™ savory crepe
Energy Index: 1.064   Protein Index: 11.941
4 servings   Change size or US/metric
Working Time: 30 minutes   15 mins prep

Crepe:
2 **eggs**
3 tablespoons **oil**
1 teaspoon **vanilla**
1 cup **skim milk**
1/2 cup **flour**
1 tablespoon **sugar**

Filling:
1/3-1/2 cup **swiss cheese** or **gruyere cheese**, shredded
1 slice **ham** (or several small slices)
1 tomato diced
dash salt
dash pepper
1 tablespoon **parsley** (optional)

1. Mix crepe ingredients together well.
2. Allow batter to sit for 30 minutes.
3. Drop 1/2 batter on skillet and medium heat for 3 min per side.
4. Lay the crepe flat on a pan or griddle over medium heat.
5. Arrange the cheese and ham on the crepe to cover the top half of the crepe.
6. Cook until the cheese is nearly all melted.
7. Spread 1/2 of the tomatoes over the cheese and ham.
8. Add salt and pepper to taste.
9. Fold the bottom half to cover the top half, then fold the right quarter over the left quarter.
10. Cook on both sides if needed.
11. Remove crepe to plate.
12. Garnish with minced parsley, if desired.

Chicken Macadamia
Energy Index: 2.059   Protein Index: 10.872
4 servings   Change size or US/metric
Working Time: 30 minutes   15 mins prep

4 **chicken breasts**
1 **avocado**
400 g   **mangoes** (1 Slice)
100 g   **macadamia nuts**
325 g   **breadcrumbs**
1 **egg**
1 tablespoon **oil**

1 Slice a pocket into Chicken Breasts.
2 Peel avocado; cut into slices; Stuff 1/4 of avocado in each chicken breast; Secure with toothpicks or netting; (Can be obtained from butchers); Can also use string.
3 Combine breadcrumbs and finely chopped macadamia nuts together.
4 In bowl, crack open egg and slightly beat egg; crumb chicken breasts.
5 Pan seal chicken; Place in oven for about 15 minutes at 180 degrees.
6 Puree Mango SLices; Pour onto plate and cut chicken breast in half; place on plate and.

Onion Pan-Fried Pork Chops.
Energy Index: 0.785   Protein Index: 10.524
2 servings   Change size or US/metric
Working Time: 10 minutes   2 mins prep

2 **pork chops**
1/2-1 cup   **all-purpose flour**
1 (2 ounces) envelope **onion soup mix**
 olive oil or **vegetable oil**

1 With your hands and onion soup mix still in sealed packet crush onions up some what, but you do not want to make

them into a powder you just want to break them up.
2. Mix flour and onion soup mix in a shallow bowl.
3. Add enough oil to bottom of a pan that would cover about half way up your pork chop.
4. Heat on medium heat until when you add flour mix to pan it sizzles.
5. Coat each pork chop with flour mixture.
6. Add to pan, about 30 seconds after adding the chops turn over, and cook until done (about 4-5 minute per side for to 3/4 inch pork chop).

Almond Chicken Vegetable Stirfry
Energy Index: 2.876   Protein Index: 9.671
4 servings
Working Time: 21 minutes 15 mins prep

2 tablespoons **vegetable oil**
1/2 teaspoon **salt**
4 ounces **bamboo shoots**
2 stalks **celery**
8 ounces **boneless skinless chicken breasts**
6 ounces **mushrooms**
1/8 **red pepper**
1 medium **onion**
1 teaspoon **gingerroot**
1 clove **garlic**
6 ounces **chicken broth**
2 teaspoons **soy sauce**
3 tablespoons **water**
2 tablespoons **cornstarch**
1/2 cup **almonds**

1. Measure and prepare all ingredients prior to beginning to cook.
2. Slice chicken breasts into bite-size pieces, set aside.
3. Drain bamboo shoots.
4. Cut celery on the bias.
5. Slice mushrooms.
6. Cut onion into 8ths- separate pieces.
7. Mince fresh gingerroot and garlic together, set aside.
8. At about 350 degrees, toast almonds for about 2 minutes.
9. Set aside.

10. Stir together the broth & soy sauce.
11. In a separate bowl, stir together the water and corn starch.
12. At medium high heat, heat oil and salt in wok until hot.
13. Add salt, stir to dissolve.
14. Stir in garlic and ginger, cook about 10 seconds.
15. If you scorch these, turn off heat, dump and re-do this step.
16. Add chicken.
17. Cook and stir until almost done, about 5 minutes.
18. Add onions, red pepper and celery, stir for about 1 minute, then add mushrooms.
19. Cook and stir another minute.
20. Add bamboo shoots.
21. Stir in broth mixture, cover and reduce heat.
22. Simmer about 3-5 minutes, or until vegetables are done.
23. Stir in water-cornstarch mixture, heat until thickened.
24. Top with toasted almonds, serve over rice.

Scrambled Eggs
Energy Index: 0.874   Protein Index: 9.810
1 servings
Working Time: 10 minutes 5 mins prep

1/2 tablespoon **butter**
3 large **eggs**
1 tablespoon **heavy cream**
1/4 teaspoon **kosher salt**
1 tablespoon snipped **fresh herbs of choice** (optional)

1. Heat 1-2 inches water in the bottom of a heavy saucepan or double boiler until just simmering- not boiling.
2. Place eggs, cream, and salt in a small mixing bowl, and with a fork, whisk until it is fairly homogenized (mass of white will start to break up), but take it easy- don't try to make whipped cream or meringue here.
3. Place a stainless mixing bowl or top of the double boiler over the water and add the butter to the pan, swirling it as it melts.
4. When the butter is completely melted, add the eggs to the pan.

You should not see instant action around the edges of the egg- if you do, your heat is way too high.

5. Don't jump right in with your spoon and stir the things to death.
6. As they start to cook, you will see curds form from the bottom.
7. Using a spoon or spatula, gently lift these curds to the top to allow the uncooked egg to flow beneath.
8. As it cooks more, it will be more a matter of lifting and folding, than stirring them briskly.
9. When the eggs are almost set (still a little wet looking), remove them from the pan, as they will cook a little more on their own.
10. If you desire smaller curds, you can chop the egg a bit and stir lightly,
11. Garnish with fresh herbs, such as chives, chervil, parsley or tarragon before serving.

Lemon Fried Chicken
Energy Index: 2.170   Protein Index: 14.991
2 servings
Working Time: 15 minutes 10 mins prep

2 **chicken breast fillets**
1/2 **lemon**
1 ounce **butter**
sea salt (optional)
fresh ground black pepper (optional)

1. Preheat a heavy-based frypan over a fairly hot flame and trim the chicken fillets, separate the tenderloins if present and set aside.
2. When the pan is hot, add the butter and melt until foaming before adding the chicken fillets.
3. After a minute or two, when the chicken has browned, turn the fillets and add the tenderloins.
4. Squeeze the juice of the lemon into the pan and cover.
5. Quarter the remains of the lemon and add to the pan, cooking for a further 5 minutes or until the juices run clear when skewered.
6. Add Sea Salt and Freshly Ground Black Pepper to taste if desired.

Kielbasa Bake
Energy Index: 2.841   Protein Index: 12.904

4 servings
Working Time: 45 minutes 15 mins prep

1 lb **kielbasa** or **Polish sausage**
1 cup roughly chopped **onions**
1 cup chopped **green peppers**
1 tablespoon **olive oil**

1. Pre-heat oven to 400F degrees.
2. In a frying pan over medium high heat fry onions and peppers until tender.
3. Slice sausage about 1/2 inch thick.
4. Fry sausage in pan with peppers and onions for 5-10 minutes.
5. Drain off excess fat.
6. Pour sausage mixture into a shallow baking dish.
7. Bake for 20-30 minutes until crispy.
8. Great served with au gratin potatoes or macaroni and cheese.

Simple Man's Bean Side Dish
Energy Index: 2.348   Protein Index: 6.185
Working Time: 5 min, Cook: 5 min.
1-1/2 lbs. canned baked beans
3/4 cup lowfat cottage cheese
3/4 cup applesauce

1. Heat beans in a microwave or in a skillet.
2. Add cottage cheese and applesauce and serve.

Grilled Ham and Cheese Sandwiches
Energy Index: 1.383   Protein Index: 7.618
Working Time: 5 min, Cook: 5 min.

1 Tbs. unsalted butter, softened
8 slices white or whole wheat bread
1 Tbs. plus 1 tsp. Dijon mustard
4 slices baked ham
4 slices fat-free Swiss cheese

1. Spread butter on one side of each piece of bread.
2. Spread mustard on unbuttered side. Place a slice of ham and a slice of cheese on mustard-coated sides of 4 slices of bread.

3. Cover with remaining bread. Place sandwiches in a heavy non-stick pan 4 over medium-high heat.
5. Cook 2 minutes per side, or until lightly toasted. Serve hot.

Tuna Fish Curry
Energy Index: 1.843   Protein Index: 13.792
Working Time: 10 min, Cook: 5 min.

1 cup water
1 cup instant rice
2 tsp. oil
1 apple, peeled and chopped
2 tsp. curry powder
1 cup tomato sauce
2 Tbs. apple juice
1/2 lb. white tuna in water, drained

1. Bring water to a boil in a saucepan over high heat.
2. Stir in rice, cover pan and remove from heat. Let stand 5 minutes.
3. Fluff with a fork. Cover and keep warm. Heat oil in a wok over medium high heat.
4. Reduce heat to medium and stir fry apple 1-2 minutes.
5. Stir in curry powder.
6. Pour in tomato sauce and bring to a boil.
7. Add juice and tuna.
8. Stir until heated throughout.
9. Serve over limited amount of rice.

Chicken Italiano
Energy Index: 4.587   Protein Index: 11.724
Working Time: 10 min, Cook: 15 min.

3 ounces angel hair pasta
1/2 lb. boneless chicken breasts, cut into thin strips
1/2 cup light Italian dressing
11 ounces frozen mixed vegetables
3-1/2 Tbs. grated Parmesan cheese, (optional)

1. Cook pasta in a large pan of boiling water 4-5 minutes until al

dente.
2. Drain.
3. Set aside and keep warm.
4. Combine chicken and 1/4 of the dressing in a heavy nonstick skillet over medium high heat.
5. Sauté chicken 2 minutes, until lightly browned.
6. Add vegetables and remaining dressing. C
7. over and simmer 7-9 minutes until vegetables are crisp tender, stirring frequently.
8. Serve over pasta.
9. Sprinkle with cheese.

Savory Chicken Squares
Energy Index: 3.717   Protein Index: 9.411
Working Time: 15 min, Cook: 20 min.

3 ounces light cream cheese, softened
2 Tbs. unsalted butter, melted
2 cups cooked chicken, cubed
2 Tbs. milk
1 Tbs. chives or scallions, chopped
1 Tbs. pimento, chopped, optional
1/2 lb. refrigerated biscuit dough

1. Preheat oven to 350°F.
2. Blend cream cheese and half the butter until smooth.
3. Add next 4 ingredients and salt and pepper to taste.
4. Mix well.
5. Separate dough into 4 rectangles and firmly press perforations around edges together to seal.
6. Spoon 1/2 cup meat mixture onto center of each rectangle.
7. Pull 4 corners of dough to top center of chicken mixture, twist slightly and seal edges.
8. Arrange on a cookie sheet. Brush tops with reserved melted butter and
9. Bake 20-25 minutes or until golden brown.

Asian Tuna
Energy Index: 0.084   Protein Index: 22.185
Working Time: 5 min, Marinate: 20 min, Cook: 10 min.

2 Tbs. plus 2 tsp. orange juice, (fresh or frozen)
1 Tbs. plus 1 tsp. sesame oil
1-1/4 tsp. sesame seeds
2 Tbs. lite soy sauce
2 tsp. fresh ginger, grated, or 1-1/4 tsp. ground ginger
2 Tbs. scallions, chopped
1 lb. tuna steak

1. In a stainless steel bowl or plastic resealable bag, combine first 6 ingredients.
2. Add the tuna and let marinate for 20 minutes.
3. Broil or grill the tuna 6 inches from the heat source for 4-5 minutes per side.
4. Cook until done as desired.

Per serving: calories 173,
fat 6.3g, 34%
calories from fat
cholesterol 53mg
protein 25.8g
carbohydrates 2.2g
fiber 0.2g
sugar 1.2g
sodium 310mg

Alaskan Crab Salad
Energy Index: 3.117   Protein Index: 10.614
Working Time: 10 min.

1 lb. european salad (or other packaged salad mix)
2 cups cherry tomatoes
1 cucumber, thinly sliced
1 lb. fancy white crabmeat
1 cup fat-free Thousand Island dressing

1. Arrange lettuce salad on plates.
2. Top with tomatoes, cucumber and crab and drizzle with dressing.

Per serving: calories 246

fat 2.0g
7% calories from fat
cholesterol 101mg
protein 26.3g
carbohydrates 30.2g
fiber 5.3g
sugar 16.1g
sodium 995mg

Grilled Tuna with Chinese Five Spice Sauce
Energy Index: 1.051   Protein Index: 19.451
Working Time: 20 min, Marinate: 30 min, Cook: 15 min.

1 lb. tuna steak
1-1/4 tsp. sesame oil
1 Tbs. plus 1 tsp. lemon juice
1/3 cup lite soy sauce
1/3 cup Hoisin sauce
2 tsp. honey
2 cloves garlic, minced
1-1/4 tsp. Chinese five spice

1. Marinate the tuna steaks in the sesame oil and lemon juice for 30 minutes.
2. Prepare an outside grill with an oiled rack set 6 inches above the heat source.
3. On a gas grill, set the heat to medium.
4. While the tuna steaks are marinating, combine the remaining sauce ingredients and heat in a pan for 10 minutes over medium heat.
5. Grill the tuna steaks for 6-7 minutes on each side, turning once, basting each side occasionally with the sauce.

Per serving: calories 205
fat 3.6g, 16% calories from fat
cholesterol 54mg
protein 26.9g
carbohydrates 15.5g
fiber 0.7g
sugar 3.0g

sodium 1098mg

Texas Chicken Burgers with Milk Gravy
Energy Index: 1.742   Protein Index: 14.529
Serves: 4
Working Time: 5 min, Cook: 10 min.

1 egg
1-1/4 lbs. ground chicken
1/4 cup plus 2 Tbs. all purpose flour
1 Tbs. unsalted butter
2 Tbs. vegetable oil
1-1/2 cups milk
1/8 tsp. hot pepper sauce

1. Beat together egg and salt and pepper to taste in a bowl until well blended.
2. Add ground chicken and mix until just combined. Form into 4 patties about 3/4 inch thick.
3. Combine 1/4 cup flour and salt and pepper to taste.
4. Dredge patties in seasoned flour.
5. Melt butter in oil in a heavy nonstick skillet over medium high heat.
6. Cook burgers about 5 minutes per side, turning once, until golden brown and chicken is just cooked through.
7. Drain burgers on paper towels and keep warm.
8. Sprinkle 2 Tbs. flour into drippings in skillet over medium heat.
9. Cook 2-3 minutes, whisking until lightly browned.
10. Whisk in milk and hot pepper sauce.
11. Increase heat to medium high and stir constantly 2-3 minutes, or until thickened.
12. Season with salt and pepper to taste and serve over chicken burgers.

Per serving: calories 389
fat 25.6g, 60% calories from fat
cholesterol 179mg
protein 29.8g
carbohydrates 8.5g
fiber 0.1g

sugar 4.5g
sodium 193mg

Steamed Whitefish Fillets
Energy Index: 0.813   Protein Index: 16.774
Working Time: 5 min, Cook: 15 min.
1-1/2 lbs. whitefish fillets
1 cup tomato juice
1 tsp. oregano
1/4 tsp. seasoned salt, or to taste
1/4 tsp. white pepper, or to taste

1 Preheat oven to 400°F.
2 Place fillets in a baking dish.
3 Combine tomato juice and seasonings in a bowl.
4 Pour over fish.
5 Cover and bake 12-18 minutes, until fish flakes easily.

Per serving: calories 151
fat 1.6g, 9% calories from fat
cholesterol 73mg
protein 30.8g
carbohydrates 2.9g
fiber 0.7g
sugar 2.1g
sodium 243mg

Italian Bean and Tuna Salad
Energy Index: 2.943   Protein Index: 17.551
Working Time: 15 min, plus refrigeration time.

11 ounces canned baby lima beans, rinsed, drained
11 ounces canned dark red kidney beans, rinsed, drained
10 ounces canned Great Northern beans, rinsed, drained
5-1/4 cherry tomatoes, cut into fourths
1/4 small cucumber, cut lengthwise into halves, seeded, sliced
3-1/2 Tbs. green or red bell pepper, chopped
1/4 red onion, thinly sliced
2 Tbs. olive oil
1/3 cup tarragon white wine vinegar

Recipes | 151

1 tsp. dried basil leaves
2 Tbs. nonfat plain yogurt
1 Tbs. lemon juice
1/2 tsp. sugar
1 Tbs. water
2 cloves garlic
11 ounces tuna steak, broiled or grilled, or canned white tuna in water, drained, flaked into small pieces
5-1/4 large lettuce leaves
2-3/4 basil or parsley sprigs

1   Combine beans, tomatoes, cucumber, pepper, and onion in large bowl.
2   Add the next 8 ingredients (basil vinaigrette) and toss.
3   Refrigerate mixture at least 4 hours for flavors to blend, stirring mixture occasionally.
4   Add tuna to mixture 1 to 2 hours before serving.
5   Spoon salad onto lettuce-lined plate; garnish with basil.

You can make the bean salad one day in advance and refrigerate, adding tuna 1 to 2 hours before serving.

Courtesy American Dry Bean Board.

Per serving: calories 454
fat 9.1g, 18% calories from fat
cholesterol 37mg
protein 36.4g
carbohydrates 59.8g
fiber 19.1g
sugar 13.3g
sodium 76mg

Ham and Cheese Chicken Turnovers
Energy Index: 1.002   Protein Index: 17.544
Working Time: 15 min, Cook: 15 min.

4 thin slices prosciutto
4 slices mozzarella cheese
4 boneless skinless chicken breast halves, pounded to 1/4 inch

thickness
toothpick
2 tsp. vegetable oil
2 tsp. unsalted butter
2 Tbs. plus 2 tsp. dry white wine
1 Tbs. plus 1 tsp. parsley, chopped

1. Place 3/4 slice of prosciutto and 3/4 slice of cheese on each flattened chicken breast.
2. Fold in half. Secure with wooden toothpicks or small skewers.
3. Heat oil and butter in a heavy nonstick skillet over medium high heat.
4. Sauté chicken turnovers 3-4 minutes per side, or until chicken is barely opaque throughout.
5. Add wine and simmer 5 minutes. Remove toothpicks before serving garnished with parsley.

Per serving: calories 351
fat 11.3g, 30% calories from fat
cholesterol 124mg
protein 50.8g
carbohydrates 7.1g
fiber 0.0g
sugar 0.1g
sodium 717mg

Beef & Cheese Burritos
Energy Index: 1.755   Protein Index: 14.552
Working Time: 10 min, Cook: 10 min.

1 lb. lean ground beef
1-1/4 cups chunky style prepared salsa
1/2 lb. cheddar cheese, cubed
8 large flour tortillas, warmed
2 cups lettuce, chopped
2 tomatoes, chopped
1/2 cup ripe olives, sliced

1. Heat a heavy nonstick skillet over medium high heat.
2. Cook beef 6-8 minutes, stirring occasionally until no longer pink.

3   Drain and discard drippings.
4   Stir in salsa and cheese.
5   Cook until cheese is melted.
6   To serve, spoon about 1/3 cup beef mixture in center of each tortilla.
7   Top with a portion of each remaining ingredient.
8   Fold bottom edge up over filling.
9   Fold sides to center, overlapping edges.

Per serving: calories 939
fat 41.4g, 40% calories from fat
cholesterol 101mg
protein 51.5g
carbohydrates 88.6g
fiber 7.0g
sugar 6.9g
sodium 1568mg

Chicken and Black Bean Sauté
Energy Index: 3.421   Protein Index: 17.952
Working Time: 10 min, Cook: 20 min.

2 tsp. unsalted butter
2/3 cup onion, finely chopped
1 lb. boneless skinless chicken breast halves, cut into 1 inch pieces
2 lbs. black beans, drained
3/4 tsp. turmeric
1/4 tsp. cayenne pepper
1/4 tsp. pepper
4 scallions, sliced
2 cups plain lowfat yogurt
4 white pitas, opened at one side and lightly toasted

1   Melt butter in a heavy nonstick skillet over medium high heat.
2   Sauté onion 5-7 minutes or until golden.
3   Add chicken and sauté 3-4 minutes or until chicken is lightly browned.
4   Stir in black beans, turmeric, cayenne and pepper and sauté 3-4 minutes.
5   Reduce heat to medium low.
6   Stir in half the scallions.

7   Sauté 2-3 minutes, stirring constantly until scallions are softened.
8   Remove from heat and stuff into pita breads.
9   Sprinkle with remaining scallions and a dollop of yogurt.

Per serving: calories 620
fat 6.9g, 10% calories from fat
cholesterol 78mg
protein 53.0g
carbohydrates 85.2g
fiber 18.9g
sugar 20.7g
sodium 704mg

Grilled Porterhouse Steaks
Energy Index: 2.118   Protein Index: 23.844
Working Time: 5 min, Cook: 10 min.

4 Porterhouse steaks, fat trimmed
 seasoned salt

1   Prepare grill or broiler.
2   Season steaks with seasoned salt and pepper to taste.
3   Grill or broil 5-6 minutes per side for medium rare meat.

Per serving: calories 454
fat 24.3g, 50% calories from fat
cholesterol 146mg
protein 54.9g
carbohydrates 0.0g
fiber 0.0g
sugar 0.0g
sodium 146mg

Quick Chicken with Lime Butter
Energy Index: 1.113   Protein Index: 19.822
Working Time: 5 min, Cook: 15 min.
6 boneless skinless chicken breast halves
3 Tbs. vegetable oil
1 lime, juiced

1/4 cup plus 2 Tbs. unsalted butter
1 Tbs. chives, minced
1 tsp. fresh dill, minced or 1/2 tsp. dried dill weed

1. Season chicken with salt and pepper to taste.
2. Heat oil in a heavy nonstick skillet over medium high heat.
3. Sauté chicken 4 minutes, or until lightly browned.
4. Turn chicken, cover pan, and reduce heat to low.
5. Cook 10 minutes, or until tender. Remove to a platter and keep warm.
6. Discard oil and wipe out pan. Add lime juice and cook over low heat until bubbly.
7. Add butter, stirring until butter becomes opaque and sauce thickens.
8. Stir in chives and dill.
9. Season with salt and pepper to taste.
10. Spoon over chicken and serve.

Per serving: calories 551
fat 30.9g, 51% calories from fat
cholesterol 205mg
protein 63.4g
carbohydrates 2.7g
fiber 0.7g
sugar 0.6g
sodium 180mg

Grilled Tuna and Bean Salad
Energy Index: 2.884   Protein Index: 18.420
Working Time: 15 min, Cook: 10 min.

4 small tuna steaks, about 3 ounces each
1 lb. canned garbanzo beans, or canned black beans
1 cup mushrooms, sliced
1 cup cherry tomatoes, halved
1/2 cup yellow bell pepper, chopped
1/4 cup red onion, chopped
1/3 cup orange juice
3 Tbs. lime juice
2 Tbs. olive oil

1 Tbs. Dijon or stoneground mustard
6 cups mixed salad greens

1. Broil tuna steaks 6 inches from heat source until fish is tender and flakes with a fork, about 5 minutes on each side.
2. Sprinkle lightly with salt and pepper.
3. While tuna is cooking, combine garbanzo beans, mushrooms, tomato, bell pepper, and onion in salad bowl.
4. In separate container, mix orange juice, lime juice, olive oil, and mustard.
5. Drizzle over the ingredients in the salad bowl.
6. Season to taste with salt and pepper.
7. Spoon salad onto serving plates and top each with a tuna steak.

Variation: If desired, you can make the salad with creamed tuna. Drain 3 ounces white tuna per serving and break into large chunks. Toss with salad mixture.

Pita Chicken Breast with Spinach
Energy Index: 3.842   Protein Index: 15.774
Working Time: 15 min, Cook: 15 min.

1 Tbs. olive oil
2 tsp. garlic cloves, coarsely chopped
4 boneless chicken breasts
1 cup red onion, thinly sliced
3 Tbs. balsamic or red wine vinegar
3 cups fresh spinach leaves
4 pita bread loaves, warm
1/3 cup feta cheese, crumbled

1. Heat oil in a heavy nonstick skillet over medium high heat.
2. Stir in garlic and salt and pepper to taste.
3. Add chicken and onion.
4. Cook 3-5 minutes per side, until chicken is golden brown.
5. Add vinegar.
6. Gradually add spinach and cook 3-4 minutes until spinach is wilted.
7. Place warm pitas on individual plates.
8. Spoon a mound of spinach on each pita and top with chicken breast.

9 Sprinkle with crumbled feta cheese and serve.

Per serving: calories 491
fat 9.7g, 18% calories from fat
cholesterol 117mg
protein 55.2g
carbohydrates 45.7g
fiber 7.7g
sugar 6.3g
sodium 756mg

Chicken Cordon Bleu
Energy Index: 2.124   Protein Index: 13.441
Serves: 4 servings

1 lb chicken breast fillets
1 tbsp honey
1 tbsp dijon mustard
1 tbsp butter
4 slices (3/4 oz each) swiss cheese
4 slices (1 oz each) boiled ham

1 Wash chicken breasts and pat dry with paper towel.
2 Pound with mallet or press under cutting board until breasts are approximately 1/2 inch thick.
3 In small mixing bowl, blend honey and mustard.
4 Dip chicken breasts in mixture to coat.
5 In large skillet, melt butter over medium heat.
6 Add chicken.
7 Cook for 4 minutes.
8 Turn.
9 Cook for 2 minutes.
10 Place one slice of ham and one slice of cheese on each chicken breast.
11 Continue cooking for 3-4 minutes.
12 Remove from pan and serve while hot.

protein - 38g –

carbohydrate 6g

Chicken Swisse
Energy Index: 1.964   Protein Index: 14.534
Serves: 4

2 thin slices reduced fat Swiss cheese
4 (4 oz each) chicken cutlets (or pounded breasts)
2 tbsp all-purpose flour
1/2 tsp black pepper
1 tbsp butter
1/2 cup chicken broth
1/4 cup dry white wine
1/4 tsp dried oregano

1   Cut each cheese slice in half to make 4 slices.
2   Place 1 cheese slice each on top of each chicken cutlet.
3   Starting at the short end, tightly roll the cutlets (jelly-roll fashion).
4   Tie each roll securely with string.
5   In flat casserole or deep plate, combine flour and pepper.
6   Mix well with fork.
7   Add cutlets and roll to coat.
8   In large non-stick skillet, melt butter over medium heat.
9   Add cutlets.
10   Turn frequently until browned on all sides (about 3 minutes).
11   Add broth, wine, and oregano to skillet.
12   Turn heat to medium-high.
13   Bring to a boil.
14   Reduce heat to medium-low.
15   Simmer until chicken is cooked through and sauce thickens.
16   Place on serving platter.
17   Cut and remove strings.
18   Serve while hot.

Crustless Easy Quiche
Energy Index: 2.667   Protein Index: 10.444
Serves: 5

1 tbsp butter or margarine
1/2 cup onion (minced)
1 cup whole kernel corn

1/2 cup cooked ham (diced)
3 tbsp green bell pepper (diced)
3 tbsp red bell pepper (diced)
2 green onions (white part only, diced)
3 eggs
1-1/2 cups whipping cream (scalded)
1/2 cup Monterey Jack cheese (shredded)

1. Preheat oven to 300 degrees.
2. In medium saucepan, heat butter.
3. Add onion.
4. Saute until tender.
5. Stir in ham, corn, green pepper, red pepper, and onions.
6. Saute until liquid has evaporated.
7. Spray a 10" glass baking dish (round) with non-stick cooking spray.
8. Pour saute mixture into baking dish.
9. In mixing bowl, beat eggs lightly.
10. Add 1/2 of scalded, hot cream.
11. Beat well.
12. Pour mixture into pan with scalded cream.
13. Stir in cheese until well-blended.
14. Pour over saute mixture in baking dish.
15. Set baking dish into larger oven-safe pan.
16. Add 1 cup boiling water to outer pan being careful not to get water into baking dish.
17. Bake for 45 minutes or until knife inserted in center comes out clean.
18. Remove from oven and let set for 5 minutes.
19. Garnish with fresh bell pepper slices and tomato wedges, if desired.

Polynesian Steaks
Energy Index: 2.808   Protein Index: 16.874

4 (8oz each) New York strip steaks (1" thick)
1/2 cup soy sauce
2 tsp ginger (minced)
2 cloves garlic (minced)
1 shallot (chopped)
1/4 tsp red pepper flakes

1/2 tsp curry powder
2 tbsp orange marmalade
4 pineapple slices (canned or fresh)

1. Trim excess fat from steaks.
2. Place steaks in shallow, glass baking dish.
3. In medium mixing bowl, combine soy sauce, ginger, garlic, shallot, red pepper, curry powder, and marmalade.
4. Mix well.
5. Pour mixture over steaks.
6. Place dish in refrigerator for 4 hours, turning steaks twice during marinading time.
7. Heat charcoal or gas grill to medium-hot.
8. Place steaks on grill 5 inches from heat.
9. Cook 12-15 minutes on each side or until done as desired.
10. Brush steaks with marinade during cooking.
11. Remove steaks from grill to serving plates.
12. Top with pineapple rings.
13. Serve while hot.

Turkey Creole-Style
Energy Index: 0.224   Protein Index: 20.741

1 boneless turkey loin (about 1-1/2 lbs)
1 dash salt
1 dash black pepper
1 tbsp butter
1 can (8 oz) stewed tomatoes
1/4 cup catsup
1 tbsp brown sugar
1 tsbp red wine vinegar
1 tsp dry mustard
1 tsp thyme (dried)
1/3 cup onion, finely chopped

1. Preheat oven to 350 degrees.
2. In a medium saucepan, combine tomatoes, catsup, brown sugar, vinegar, mustard, thyme, and onion.
3. Bring to a boil.
4. Reduce heat.
5. Simmer for 15 minutes or until sauce thickens slightly.

6. In a large skillet, melt the butter
7. Brown the turkey loin on all sides in the butter.
8. Sprinkle with salt and pepper.
9. Transfer turkey loin to a casserole or Dutch oven.
10. Pour sauce over turkey loin.
11. Cook turkey loin for about 40 minutes, turning turkey over once. Do not overcook..
12. Slice meat and serve by spooning sauce over slices.

Tahitian Tuna Steaks
Energy Index: 1.009   Protein Index: 20.191

1.5 pounds tuna steaks (1-inch thick)
1/4 cup lime juice
2 tbsp olive oil
1 tsp gingerroot (finely chopped)
1/4 tsp salt
1/4 tsp cayenne pepper
1 clove garlic (crushed)
2 limes (cut into wedges)

1. Cut tuna steaks into six serving-size pieces.
2. In shallow, non-metal baking dish, combine lime juice, olive oil, gingerroot, salt, cayenne pepper, and garlic.
3. Blend well.
4. Add tuna steaks.
5. Turn to coat.
6. Cover and refrigerate for 1-24 hours.
7. Preheat gas or charcoal grill.
8. Remove fish from marinade.
9. Reserve marinade, but transfer to small bowl.
10. Place steaks on grill four inches from heat.
11. Cook for 7-8 minutes per side, basting with marinade throughout.
12. Fish is done when it flakes easily with a fork.
13. Remove fish to serving plates.
14. Garnish with lime wedges.
15. Serve while hot.

Chicken Divan
Energy Index: 1.434   Protein Index: 15.973

4 large boneless, skinless chicken breasts
3 tbsp flour
1/4 tsp white pepper
3 tbsp butter
1 cup milk
1/4 cup swiss cheese (shredded)
2 tbsp parmesan cheese (grated)
1 pkg (10 oz) frozen broccoli spears (thawed, drained)

1. Preheat oven to 400 degrees.
2. Wash chicken breasts and pat dry with paper towel.
3. In shallow baking dish, combine 2 tbsp flour and white pepper.
4. Dip chicken breasts in flour mixture to coat evenly.
5. In large skillet, melt 2 tbsp butter over medium heat.
6. Add chicken.
7. Cook for 2 minutes.
8. Turn.
9. Cook for 2 minutes.
10. Transfer chicken to ovenproof casserole for baking.
11. Melt remaining 1 tbsp butter in skillet.
12. Stir in 1 tbsp flour.
13. Cook 1 minute.
14. Add milk.
15. Stir and cook for 2 minutes or until thickened.
16. Remove from heat.
17. Stir in cheeses.
18. Place broccoli over chicken in baking dish.
19. Pour sauce over chicken and broccoli.
20. Sprinkle with extra parmesan cheese, if desired.
21. Bake 20 minutes.
22. Serve while hot.

Indonesian Chicken Breasts
Energy Index: 2.664   Protein Index: 19.527

1/2 cup orange juice concentrate
1/4 cup peanut butter (smooth type)

2 tsps curry powder
4 boneless, skinless chicken breast halves
1/2 medium red bell pepper cut into wide strips
1/2 medium green bell pepper cut into wide strips
1/4 cup shredded, unsweetened coconut

1. Blend orange juice, peanut butter, and curry powder in mixing bowl.
2. Add chicken to marinade being sure to cover chicken entirely.
3. Cover and refrigerate mixture for at least an hour or up to 24 hours.
4. After marinading for at least one hour, remove chicken and discard marinade.
5. Grill chicken and bell peppers over charcoal or on a gas grill using medium heat.
6. Cook for 15-20 minutes or until chicken juices run clear when breasts are pierced with a fork.
7. Serve chicken with grilled pepper strips sprinkled with coconut.

Red Snapper a L'Orange
Energy Index: 2.713   Protein Index: 19.882

1-1/2 pound red snapper fillets
1/2 tsp fresh ground black pepper
2 tbsp orange juice
1 tsp orange rind
3 tbsp olive oil
1/2 tsp nutmeg
1 large orange (thinly sliced)

1. Preheat oven to 350 degrees.
2. In small mixing bowl, combine pepper, juice, rind, and oil.
3. Blend well.
4. Spray baking dish with non-stick cooking spray.
5. Arrange fillets in baking dish.
6. Drizzle sauce over fish.
7. Sprinkle with nutmeg.
8. Place on center rack of oven.
9. Bake for 20-30 minutes or until fish flakes easily with fork.

10   Remove to serving plates.
11   Garnish with fresh orange slices.
12   Serve while hot.

Thai Pork Salad
Energy Index: 4.811   Protein Index: 17.423
Serves: 4

1/2 lb lean pork strips (cooked, cut into cubes, chilled)
8 cups mixed salad greens including Chinese cabbage (torn into bite-size pieces)
1 medium avocado (halved, seeded, peeled, cubed)
1 large carrot (julienned)
1/4 cup green onions (sliced)
1/4 cup peanuts or honey-roasted peanuts
1/2 cup fat free Italian dressing
1 tbsp soy sauce
1-1/2 tsp fresh ginger (grated)
1/2 tsp crushed red pepper flakes

1   Distribute salad greens on four dinner plates.
2   Arrange pork cubes, avocado cubes, and carrots.
3   In small mixing bowl, combine Italian dressing, soy sauce, ginger, and red pepper.
4   Blend well.
5   Drizzle dressing over prepared salads.
6   Top each salad with green onions and peanuts.
7   Serve cold.

Polynesian Mango Shrimp Kebobs
Energy Index: 3.771   Protein Index: 10.842
Serves: 6

1/3 cup lemon juice
1 tbsp dry ground mustard
1 tbsp olive oil
1 tsp ground cumin
1/2 tsp ground coriander

1/2 tsp salt
1/8 tsp paprika
1.5 pounds uncooked, large shrimp (peeled, deveined)
2 limes (cut into wedges)
1 medium mango (cut into 1-inch cubes)

1. In large casserole or other dish combine lemon juice, mustard, oil, cumin, coriander, salt, and paprika.
2. Add shrimp.
3. Toss to coat.
4. Cover and refrigerate for 1-4 hours.
5. Preheat gas or charcoal grill.
6. Remove shrimp from marinade.
7. Reserve marinade, but transfer to smaller bowl.
8. Thread shrimp and mango onto six metal skewers, leaving a small space between each piece.
9. Place kebobs on grill 5-6 inches from heat and close cover.
10. Grill about 10 minutes, turning 2-3 times and brushing with leftover marinade.
11. Shrimp are done when they are pink and firm.
12. Discard remaining marinade.
13. Remove kebobs from skewers onto six serving plates.
14. Garnish with lime wedges.

Glossary

adinosine triphosphate
the molecule needed to produce chemical reactions during exercise.

apnea
condition in which the sufferer stops breathing for 10 seconds or longer, 5 to 50 times an hour. Apnea is offened experienced during sleep and can be caused by obesity, alcohol, and enlarged nasal tissue among other causes. Effects of apnea can include poor sleep, hypertension, and heart disease.

Artificially Extreme Food (AEF)
any man-made food that is highly concentrated (usually involving sugars), and thus, unnatural in its effects on the human body. AEFs are often found in heavily processed foods and at fast food restaurants, but can also be extremely concentrated natural foods. They include doughnuts, espresso, and orange juice.

ATP
adinosine triphosphate.

basal metabolism
the basic processes of maintaining life like breathing, maintaining body temperature, pumping blood, etc.

basal metobolic rate (BMR)
the rate at which your body burns calories doing basic life-sustaining activities.

Building Materials
amino acids that cells need in order to operate. These building materials can be found mostly in proteins and should eaten after exercise.

calorie
the unit of energy that is contained in any substance. Calories usually refer to 1000 calories and are actually kilocalories. A can of cola with 200 calories actually has 200,000 calories or 200 kilocalories. For the purposes of this book, we refer to kilocalories as calories.

carbohydrate
a structural component of living cells and a source of energy for animals. Simple sugars like table sugar and corn syrup, and complex carbohydrates like starch are all carbohydrates.

carnivore
strictly a meat eater.

cholesterol	a type of fat that animals make (humans included) in their liver. Low-density lipoprotein cholesterol (LDL) is the bad cholesterol and is one of the main causes of heart disease in Western culture. Below 130 mg/dL is optimal for most people. High-density lipoprotein (HDL) is the good guy because high levels of it in the bloodstream seem to prevent heart disease. Above 40 mg/dL is optimal.
Culture-less Human	a theoretical human who has no cultural ties instructing him how to live and how to eat. People today cannot be removed from culture, but the culture-less human is a tool that shows how we are designed to eat.
dietary fiber	any complex carbohydrate that human bodies cannot digest. Cellulose is a common form of fiber and is usually found in leafy vegetables. Natural Man's diet was full of dietary fiber, but modern diets are generally deficient in the substance.
digestive tract	the area in an animal's body that alters food into something that can be used by the body's cells.
Energy	the substance needed to complete basic life functions. Energy is contained in everything, but humans get our energy from the food we eat. Energy is measured in calories.
essential amino acid	any amino acid that the body cannot produce on its own and is needed in basic life functions.
essential fatty acid	a fatty acid that is required by the body to opperate normally.
The Evolution Diet	the plan of eating in a manner human bodies were designed to eat. This involves eating many small portions of low-sugar, high-fiber foods throughout the day and before exercise and a large high-protein meal after exercise and before rest and sleep.
The Evolution Plan	see The Evolution Diet
exercise	physical activity for the benefit of one's body. Culture-less humans exercised by hunting and gathering among other means.

Glossary | 169

fat   a soft greasy substance found in animal tissue and consisting of a mixture of lipids (mostly triglycerides). Fat contains 9 kilocalories per gram and is easier to digest than protein, but more difficult than carbohydrates. Fat can be found in 4 forms: saturated (solid at room temperature and found mainly in animal products, butter), monounsaturated (liquid at room temperature and found in olive oil), polyunsaturated (liquid at room temprature and found in vegetable oils), cholesterol (solid and found in animal products).

fatty acid   any of a class of aliphatic monocarboxylic acids that are part of a lipid molecule. Fatty acids the free fat molecules that are found in the bloodstream. Some fatty acids are essential to good health because they aid in the digestion of vitamins.

frugivore   an animal that usually eats fruit and sometimes eats other plants or small animals.

ghrelin   peptide hormone that has a significant impact on one's appetite by increasing hunger when heavily present in the bloodstream.

glycemic index   an extremely flawed gauge of the energy potential of a particular food. The Glycemic index shows how much a particular food will increase a person's blood sugar level.

glycemic load   the rate at which a particular food affects one's blood sugar with regard to its density.

HCl   hydrochloric acid. This acid is present in the stomach and breaks down the food we eat. The presence of HCl in the stomach can be alterred based on what foods we eat- the more protein we eat, the higher the amount of acid is released. The more acid in the stomach, the lower the pH level. pH=1 is extremely acidic, while pH=14 is extremely basic.

herbivore   strictly a plant eater.

hunter-gatherer society	social structure for humans before agriculturization. Clans of people would roam for location to location eating the available plantlife (gathering), and hunting nearby animals. This style of living was the norm for humans for 100,000 years before civilizations began. Humans evolved to fit this lifestyle perfectly and are still designed to live that way
hyperglycemia	abnormally high blood sugar usually associated with diabetes.
hypertension	a common disorder in which blood pressure remains abnormally high (a reading of 140/90 mm Hg or greater).
hypoglycemia	abnormally low blood sugar usually resulting from excessive insulin or a poor diet. The Evolution Diet prevents this by encouraging a balanced level of energy throughout the day.
kilocalorie	1000 calories.
leptin	hormone that is increased with the increased presence of fat and tells the brain that the person is full.
Life Process Facilitators	vitamins and minerals needed for a perfectly healthy life.
LoS Hi-Fi Foods	low sugar hi fiber foods, generally consisting of complex carbohydrates with minimal amounts of protein and fats. These foods should be eaten often in low amounts throughout the day, after a small breakfast and before a large high-protein dinner.
low-carb diet	any method of eating that limits the intake of carbohydrates to unnatural porportions. These diets are used, mainly, to take weight off, but also reduce energy and increase the amount of toxins within the body. Some have said this style of eating, "bores us to weight loss."
Natural Man	human kind that does not rely on processed foods. This is a theoretical tool used to illustrate exactly how we should be eating.
omnivore	an animal that eats both meat and plant foods.

Glossary

oral cavity — the area in an animal's digestive system where the food enters. Carnivores have sharp teeth, herbivores generally have flat teeth.

protein — any of the nitrogenous organic compounds that are vital for living cells. Proteins contain amino acids, some essential for life. Energy can also be derived from protein when needed through protein metabolism. Protein can be found in meats, dairy, eggs, fish, and some vegetables.

serotonin — a neurotransmitter that has a calming effect on humans and naturally lowers brain activity.

sleep apnea — transient cessation of respiration during sleep. This is usually caused by obesity, alcohol use, some pharmaceuticals, or poor diet. The result is poor sleep, high blood toxicity, and lower BMR, among other symptoms.

tryptophan — an amino acid that can be found in many animal proteins. It aids the body in production of niacin, which helps produce serotonin, a natural sedative.

vasoconstriction — the process in which blood vessels constrict to limit the blood flow to a particular area of the body.

vasodilation — dilation of the blood vessels (especially the arteries) in order to allow more blood to flow to a particular area of the body.

Notes

The Purpose of a Diet

Yo-yo Dieting: http://www.healthday.com/view.cfm?id=511643. *Genes*: Britton 2004; http://news.nationalgeographic.com/news/2002/09/0924_020924_dnachimp.html. *Obesity*: ttp://www.healthinsite.gov.au/content/internal/page.cfm?ObjID=000333EF-EC5C-1E1C-940083032BFA006D. *Fewer genes*: http://txtwriter.com/Onscience/Articles/fewgenes.html. *How food works*: http://home.howstuffworks.com/food.htm

Digestive Tract

Eat Our Colors: *Health* magazine, April 2004. *Stomach acidity*: http://www.smartskincare.com/skinbiology/sebum.html. *Decreased oral health*: Larsen 1998. *Scissor-like motion*: Klein 1999:204. *Chimps*: Harris 1989:37-38. *Dogs are color blind*: http://www.uwsp.edu/psych/dog/LA/DrP4.htm. *Stomach acidity*: http://www.smartskincare.com/skinbiology/sebum.html. *Digestive system*: http://digestive.niddk.nih.gov/ddiseases/pubs/yrdd/index.htm. *Animals' digestive tract*: http://www.hillstrath.on.ca/moffatt/bio3a/digestive/vartheme.htm

The Cultureless Diet

Neotame: http://www.neotame.com/about.asp. *Disgusting Foods*: D'Amato, Erik. 1998. *African insect food*: http://www.si.edu/resource/faq/nmnh/buginfo/inasfood.htm

What A Cultureless Person Would Eat

Sedentary lifestyle: Larsen, 1995; *Fermentation*: Rush, 2000; Chivers, 1994:60-64. *Grains*: Kushi, 1993. *Mastodons*: http://www.unmuseum.org/missingm.htm

Carbohydrate Is Not A Four Letter Word

Quote: http://www.yalemedicalgroup.org/news/ymg_archive.html. *High Fiber*: http://www.healthcastle.com/candiettx_08_02.shtml

What Too Much Sugar Does To Us

Diabetes: http://diabetes.about.com/library/blnews/blnobesityenzyme1201.htm, http://my.webmd.com/hw/diabetes_1_2/uq1444.asp?lastselectedguid={5FE84E90-BC77-4056-A91C-9531713CA348}. *Quote*: Rush, 2000. *Islets of Langerhans*: http://www.medterms.com/script/main/art.asp?articlekey=4054. *Blood sugar*: http://www.prosperityplace.com/bdy_mind/bldsgar.html. *Snickers*: http://www.mmmars.com/cai/snickers/faq.html

We Are Made of Proteins

Protein: Harris 1989:306-7. *Protein Metabolism*: http://www.trans4mind.com/personal_development/nutrition/stress/BodyStress.htm, http://insulin-pumpers.org/howto/pfandbs-2.html

With Friends Like Fats, Who Needs Enemies

Cholesterol: http://www.americanheart.org/presenter.jhtml?identifier=180. *Trans fats/partially hydrogenated oils*: http://www.recoverymedicine.com/hydrogenated_oils.htm

Eat Foods When You Would Naturally Eat Them

Toxicity: http://www.anyvitamins.com/vitamin-c-ascorbicacid-info.htm

Avoid Intake of Artificially Extreme Foods

Coffee: http://www.meinl.com/CoffeeService/quality/facts.htm; http://magma.nationalgeographic.com/ngm/0501/feature1/. *Tortilla Chips*: http://my.webmd.com/content/pages/7/3220_282.htm?printing=true#2. *World Obesity*: http://www.bbc.co.uk/apps/ifl/skillswise/gigaquiz?path=inthe-news/2003/0123&infile=0123&pool=numbers10

Caffeine: J.J. Barone, H.R. Roberts: 1996:119-129. *Caffeine content*: http://www.cspinet.org/new/cafchart.htm

Basal Metabolism

BMR: http://www.thedietchannel.com/Weight loss3.htm. *BMR and breathing*: http://www.encyclopedia.com/html/m1/metabolism.asp

The Importance of Exercise

Exercise expenditure: http://www.netfit.co.uk/fatcal.htm.

Breathing and Sleep

Sleep Foods: Sears 2002

Stress

Stress and Sleep: http://www.annecollins.com/weight-loss-support/stress-overweight.htm. *Stress and Weight loss*: http://www.annecollins.com/weight-loss-support/stress-overweight.htm.

Bibliography

Abrams, H.L. 1987. "The Preference for Animal Protein and Fat: A Cross-Cultural

Surkey." In *Food and Evolution: Toward a Theory of Human Food Habits*, ed. Marvin Harris and Eric Ross, 207-223. Philadelphia: Temple University Press.

Ardrey, Robert. 1961. *African Genisis: A Personal Investigation into the Animal Origines and Nature of Man*. New York: Atheneum.

Ascherio, Alberto, M. D. 1999. *Trans Fatty Acids and Coronary Heart Disease*. The New England Journal of Medicine.

Aubert, Claude, and Pierre Frapa. 1985. *Hunger and Health*. Emmaus, Penn.: Rodale Press.

Baksh, Michael. 1985. "Faunal Food as a 'Limiting Factor' on Amazonian Cultural Behavior: A Machiguenga Example." *Research in Economic Anthropology* 7:145-175.

Barone, J. J., H. R. Roberts (1996) "Caffeine Consumption." *Food Chemistry and Toxicology*, vol. 34, pp. 119-129

Barzun, Jacques. 2000. *From Dawn to Decadence*. New York: HarperCollins Publishers.

Beadle, G. 1981. "The Ancestor of Corn." *Scientific American* 242(1):96-103

Benedict, Ruth. 1934. *Patterns of Culture*. Boston: Houghton Miffin.

Bouchez, Collett. "Yo-Yo Dieting Tugs on Your Heart's Strings." *Health Day* [Online] Available: http://www.healthday.com/view.cfm?id=511643

Bowen, R. "Ghrelin." [Online] Available http://arbl.cvmbs.colostate.edu/hbooks/pathphys/endocrine/gi/ghrelin.html May 1, 2005.

Braidwood, Linda, and R. Braidwood. 1986. "Prelude to the Appearance of Village-Farming Communities in Southwestern Asia." In *Ancient Anatolia: Aspects of Change and Cultural Development*, ed. J. V. Canby et al., 3-11 Madison, Wis.: University of Wisconsin Press.

Brain, C. K. 1981. *The Hunters or the Hunted*. Chicago: University of Chicago Press.

Brody, Jane E. 1988. "It's Not Just the Calories, It's Their Source." *New York Times*, July 12, C3

Buchbinder, G. 1997. "Nutritional Stress and Post-Contact Population Decline Among the Maring of New Guinea." In *Malnutrition, Behavior, and Social Organization*, ed. L.S. Greene, 109-147. New York: Academic press.

Campbell, Bernard. 1985. *Human Evolution: An Introduction to Man's Adaption*. Hawthorne, N.Y.: Aldine de Gruyter.

Carrier, David. 1984. "The Energetic Paradox of Human Running and Hominid

Evolution." *Current Anthropology* 25:483-495.

Chagnon, Napoleon, and R. Hames. 1979. "Protein Deficiency and Tribal Warfare in Amazonia: New Data." *Science* 203:910-913.

Chang, Te-Tzu. 1983. "The Origins and Early Culture of the Cereal Grains and Food Legumes." In *The Origins of Chinese Civilization*, ed. David Knightley, 65-94. Berkley: University of California Press.

Chivers, D. 1994. "Diet and Guts." In *Cambridge Encyclopedia of Human Evolution*, ed. Steve Jones, Robert Martin, and David Pilbeam, New York: Cambridge University Press, 60-64.

Cohen, Mark. 1977. *The Food Crisis in Prehistory*. New Haven: Yale University Press.

Cohen, Mark, and George Armelagos, eds. 1984. *Paleopathology and the Origin of Agriculture*. New York: Academic Press.

Cowart, B. 1981. "Development of Taste Perception in Humans." *Psychological Bulletin* 90:43-73.

Dennet, G. and J. Connell. 1988. "Acculturation and Health in the Highlands of Papua new Guinea," *Current Anthropology* 29:273-199.

Denton, D. A. 1982. *The Hunger for Salt*. New York: Springer Verlag.

D'Amato, Erik. 1998 "The mystery of disgust - reflections on what disgusts people - includes related articles." *Psychology Today*. Jan-Feb 1998.

Draper, Patricia, and Nancy Howell. 2002 Nutritional status of !Kung children. Conference on Hunting and Gathering Societies, Edinburgh, Scotland, 2002.

Dreaon, Darlene M. et al. 1988. "Dietary Fat: Carbohydrate Ratio and Obesity in Middle-Aged men." *American Journal of Clinical Nutrition* 47:995-1000.

Dufour, Darna. 1986. "Insects as Food: A Case Study from the Northwest Amazon." *American Anthropologist* 89:383-397.

Dyets. "Typical Caloric Density Information." [Online] Available: http://www.dyets.com/caloric.htm

Eldredge, Niles, and Ian Tattersall. 1982. *The Myths of Human Evolution*. New York: Columbia University Press.

Estioko-Griffin, Agnes, and P. B. Griffin. 1981. "Woman the Huner: The Agata." In *Woman the Gatherer*, ed. Frances Dahlberg, 121-151. Ñew Haven: Yale University Press.

Ford, R. 1979. "Gathering and Gardening: Trends and Consequences of Hopewell Subsistence Strategies." In *Hopewell Archaeology: The Chilliocothe*

Conference, ed. D. S. Brose and N. Greber, 234-238. Kent, Ohio: Kent State University Press.

Geertz, C. 1963. *Agricultural Involution*. Berkley: University of California Press.

Good, Kenneth. 1987. "Limiting Factors in Amazonian Ecology." In *Food and Evolution: Toward a Theory of Human Feed Habits*, ed. M. harris and E. Ross, 407-426. Philadelphia: Temple University Press.

Goodman, Alan H., R.B. Thomas, A. C. Swedlund, and G. Armelagos. 1988. "Biocultural Perspectives on Stress in Prehistoric, and Contemporary Population Research ." *Yearbook of Physical Anthropology* 31:169-202.

Gould, Richard. 1982. "To Have and Not to Hace: The Ecology of Sharing Among Huner-Gatherers." In *Resourse MAnagers: North American and Australian Hunter-Gatherers*, ed. Nancy Williams and Eugene Hunn, 69-91. Boulder, Colo.: Westview Press.

Gramby, R. 1977. "Deerskins and Hunting Territories: Competition for a Scarce Resource of the Northeastern Woodlans." American Antiquity 42:601-605.

Greensberg, Joseph C., Christy Turner, and S. Zegura. 1986. "The Settlement of the Americas: A Comparison of the Linguistic, Dental and Genetic Evidence." *Current Anthropology* 28:647.

Gumbel, Peter. 1988. "Down on the Farm: Societs Try Once More to Straighten Out Old Agricultural Mess." *Wall Street Journal,* Dec. 2, 1.

Hamilton, William. 1987. "Omnivorous Primate Diets and Human Over-Consumption of Meat." In *Food and Evolution: Toward a Theory of Human Feed Habits*, ed. M. harris and E. Ross, 407-426. Philadelphia: Temple University Press.

Hansen, J. D. L. 1993. Hunter-gatherer to pastoral way of life: Effects of the transition on health, growth, and nutritional status. Southern African Journal of Science 89:559-564.

Harding, Robert. 1975. "Meat Eating and Hunting in Baboons." In *Socioecology and Psychology of Primates, ed. R. H. Tuttle*, 245-257. The Hague: Mouton.

Harris, David. 1987. "Aboriginal Subsistence in a Tropical Rain Forest Environment: Food Procurement, Cannibalism and Population Regulation in Northeastern Australia." In *Food and Evolution: Toward a Theory of Human Feed Habits*, ed. M. harris and E. Ross, 407-426. Philadelphia: Temple University Press.

Harris, Marvin. 1985. *Good to Eat: Riddles of Food and Culture*. New York: Simon and Schuster.

Harris, Marvin. 1989. *Our Kind*. New York: Harper & Row, Publishers, Inc.

Hayden, Brian. 1986. "Resources, Rivalry and Reproduction: The Influence of Basic Resourse Characteristics on Reproductive Behavior." In *Culture and*

Reproduction: An Anthropological Critique of Demographic Transition Theory, ed. W. P. Handwerker, 176-195. Boulder, Colo.: Westview Press.

Hayden, Brian, M Eldridge, A. Eldridge, and A. Cannon. 1985. "Complex Hunter-Gatherers in Interior British Columbia." In *Prehistoric Hunter-Gatherers: The Emergence of Cultural Complexity*, ed. D. Price and J. Brown, 181-199. New York: Academic Press.

Heath, R. G., ed. 1964. *The Role of Pleasure in Behavior.* New York: Harper & Roq, Publishers.

Henry, Donald. 1985. "Preagricultural Sedentism: The Natufian Example." In *Prehistoric Hunter-Gatherers: The Emergence of Cultural Complexity*, ed. D. Price and J. Brown, 365-381. New York: Academic Press.

Hiraiwa-Hasegawa, M., et al. 1986. "Aggression Toward Large Carnivores by Wild Chimpanzees of Mahale Mountains Nation Park, Tanzania." *Folia Primatologica* 47(1):8-13.

Jenike, M. R. 1989. "Seasonal Hunger Among Tropical Africans: The Lese Case." *American Journal of Physical Anthropology* 78:247.

Karoda, S. 1984. "Interaction over Food Among Pygmy Chimpanzees." In *The Pygmy Chimpanzee*, ed. R. L. Susman, 301-324. New York: W. W. Norton.

Klein, R. 1999. *The Human Career: Human Biological and Cultural Origins*, 2nd edition. Chicago: University of Chicago Press.

Leavitt, Gregory. 1977. "!Kung Bushman Subsistence: An Inpit-Output Analysis." In *Environment and Cutural Behavior*, ed. A. O. Vayda, 47-79. Garden City, N.Y.: Natural History Press.

Lewin, Roger. 1984. "Man the Scavenger." *Science* 224:861-862.

Lewontin, R., S. Rose, and L. Kamin. 1984. *Not in Our Genes: Biology, Ideology and Human Nature.* New York: Pantheon.

Lieverman, Leslie. 1987. "Biocultural Consequences of Animals Versus Plants As Sources of Gat, and Other Nutrients." *Food and Evolution: Toward a Theory of Human Feed Habits*, ed. M. harris and E. Ross, 225-258. Philadelphia: Temple University Press.

Lizot, Jaques. 1979. "On Food Taboos and Amazon Cultural Ecology." *Current Anthropology* 20:150-151.

McGrew, W. C. 1987. "Toos to Get Food: The Subsistence of Tasmanian Aborigines and Tanzanian Chimpanzees Compared." *Journal of Anthropological Research* 43:247-258.

Maclachlan, Morgan. 1983. *Why They Did Not Starve: Biocultural Adaption is a South Indian Village.* Philadelphia: Institute for the Study of Human Issues.

Martin, Roy, and Barbara Mullen. 1987. "Control of Good Intake: Mechanisms and Consequences." *Nutrition Today*, Sept./Oct., 4-10.

Morse, E. Robert. 2002. *Amazement*. Lincoln, NE: iUniverse.

Morwood, Mike, Thomas Sutikna, and Richard Roberts. "The People Time Forgot." *National Geographic*. April, 2005: p. 2.

National Womens's Health Resource Centers. "Stress: Treatment" [Online] Available: http://health.ivillage.com/mindbody/mbstress/0,,nwhrc_75hm0msw,00.html?iv_arrivalSA=1&iv_cobrandRef=0&iv_arrival_freq=1&pba=adid=16657989, May 1, 2005.

Nishida, Toshisada. 1973. "The Ant-Gathering Behavior by the Use of Tools Among Wild Chimpanzees of the Mahale Mountains." *Journal of Human Evolution* 2:357-370.

Pennington, Renee, and Henry Harpending. 1988. "Fitness and Fertility Among Kalahari !Kung." *American Journal of Physical Anthropology* 77-303-319.

Price, Douglas, and James Brown, eds. 1985. Prehistoric Hunter-Gatherers: *The Emergence of Cultural Complexity*. New York: Academic Press.

Reid, T. R. "Caffeine." *National Geographic*. January, 2005: p.2.

Rotberg, Robert, and Theodore Rebb. 1985. Hunger and History: *The Impact of Changing Food Production and Consumption Patterns on Society*. New York: Cambridge University Press.

Rozin, P., and D. schiller. 1980. "The Nature and Acquisition of a Preference for Chili Peppers by Humans." *Motication and Emotion* 4:77-101.

Rush, John A. "Applying Medical Anthropology: Gut Morphology, Cultural Eating Habits, Digestive Failure, and Ill Health." [Online] Available: http://www.medanth.org/case_studies/rush01.htm

Ruskin, Jeremy. 2003. "The fast food trap: how commercialism creates overweight children - Special Report: Kids and Corporate Culture." *Mothering*. Nov-Dec 2003.

Shipman, Pat. 1986. "Scavenging or Hunting in Early Hominids: Theoretical Framework and Tests." *American Anthropologist* 88:27-43.

Sims, E., and E. Danforth. 1987. "Expenditure and Storage of Enrgy in Man." In *Ancestors: Clinical Investigation* 79:1019-1025.

Sorokin, Pitirm. 1975. *Hunger as a Factor in Human Affairs*. Gainsville, Fla.: University Presses of Florida.

Speth, J. 1987. "Early Hominid Subsistence Strategies in Seasonal Habitats." *Journal of Archaeological Science* 14:13-29.

Stahl, Ann. 1984. "Hominid Dietary Selection Before Fire." *Current Anthropology* 25:151-168.

Tanner, Nancy. 1983. "Hunters, Gatherers, and Sex Toles in Space and Time." *American Anthropologist* 85:335-341.

Testat, Alain. 1982. "The Significance of Food-Storage Among Hunter-Gatherers: Residence Patterns, Population Densities and Social Inequalities." Current Anthropology 23:523-537.

Warner, Jennifer. "Skinny Smokers Just As Unhealthy." [Online] Available: http://my.webmd.com/content/article/24/1837_50611.http://my.webmd.com/content/article/24/1837_50611.htm

Waterlow, J. C. 1986. "Metabolic Adaption to Low Intakes of Energy and Protein." *Annual Review of Nutrition* 6:495.

Wilmsen, E. T. 1982. "Studies in diet, nutrition, and fertility among a group of Kalahari Bushmen in Botswana." Social Science Information 21(1):95-125.